The
Body
Fat
BREAKTHROUGH

The
Body
Fat
BREAKTHROUGH

Tap the Muscle-Building Power of Negative Training and Lose Up to

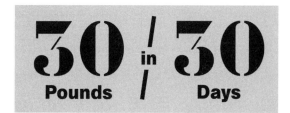

30 *in* **30**
Pounds / **Days**

Ellington Darden, PhD

RODALE.

Exclusive direct mail hardcover published simultaneously in April 2014 by Rodale Inc.

© 2014 by Ellington Darden, PhD

Rodale books may be purchased for business or promotional use or for special sales.
For information, please write to:
Special Markets Department, Rodale Inc., 733 Third Avenue, New York, NY 10017.

Men's Health is a registered trademark of Rodale Inc.

Printed in the United States of America

Rodale Inc. makes every effort to use acid-free ∞, recycled paper ♻.

Illustrations by Keelan Parham

Exercise photographs by Thomas MacDonald; other photographs, including before-and-after
photographs, by Ellington Darden and Mindy Miller, with the exception of Inga Cook (page 48);
Scott LeGear (page 54); Mats Thulin (pages 64, 310); Philip Schwartz (page 105);
and William Boyd (pages 308, 309)

Book design by Mike Smith

Library of Congress Cataloging-in-Publication Data is on file with the publisher.
ISBN-13: 978–1–62336–103–7 trade hardcover

Distributed to the trade by Macmillan
2   4   6   8   10   9   7   5   3   1   trade

We inspire and enable people to improve their lives and the world around them.
rodalebooks.com

Picture the Possibilities
Do for yourself what these people have achieved.

. . . .

Built a Brand-New Body

"Dr. Darden's program changed my life. I eat better, I drink more water, and I exercise harder. I'm a much healthier person with a brand-new body."
—ERIKA GREENE (SEE PAGE 8)

Dropped 80 Pounds in 80 Days

"I lost 80 pounds in the first 80 days. It was unbelievable, absolutely unbelievable!"
—BOB SMITH (SEE PAGE 22)

Trimmed 12 Inches off Waist

"I burned multiple layers of fat from my waist and am stronger and more fit than ever."
—MELISSA NORMAN (SEE PAGE 38)

Created Best Shape Ever

"The Breakthrough program has given me the tools to get back to my high-school body weight and I'm now in the best shape of my life."
—STORM ROBERTS (SEE PAGE 76)

Added Curves in the Right Places

"Off came the pounds and inches. Dr. Darden's unique negative training sharpened all my curves."
—ASHLEY MEISNER (SEE PAGE 16)

Recognized for Muscularity

"A muscular body—I've always wanted one for as long as I can remember. During the after-12-week measurements, Dr. Darden told me that my muscularity was the best of any man who finished his Breakthrough program. My self-confidence is now at an all-time high."
—AUSTIN DEELY (SEE PAGE 186)

. . . .

Before-and-after photos of these participants in the Body Fat Breakthrough program, and many others, appear throughout this book.

CONTENTS

ANGEL RODRIGUEZ
BEFORE & AFTER

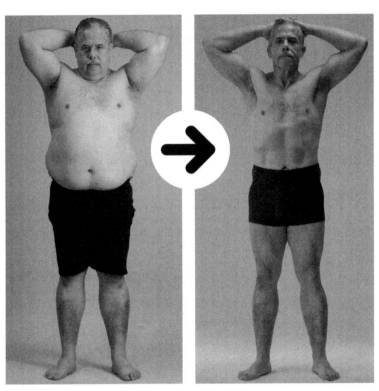

AGE 48, HEIGHT 5'8"

BEFORE BODY WEIGHT

281.5
POUNDS

AFTER BODY WEIGHT

181
POUNDS

AFTER 30 WEEKS

121
POUNDS OF FAT LOSS

20.125
INCHES OFF WAIST

20.5
POUNDS OF MUSCLE GAIN

A New and Better Body

Your friends and family won't recognize you

WHEN Angel Rodriguez knocked on his mother's back door, she quickly retreated from the entrance and walked into the main part of the house. She didn't recognize her son of 48 years.

"Mom, it's me, Angel."

Rodriguez hadn't visited his mother, who was living in Miami, in 7 months. In that time, he had lost 121 pounds of fat, taken 20 inches off his waist, and put on 20.5 pounds of solid muscle. He looked nothing like her big-bellied son. She thought he might be an intruder, and a well-muscled one at that. For a moment, she considered calling the cops.

"I hesitated for a few seconds," says Rodriguez, "then I knocked louder and yelled, 'Mom, mom!' . . . and grinned at her in my special way."

Then it clicked and she responded in her Cuban accent, *"Angel, me parece mentira.* [I can't believe it.] What have you done to yourself?"

What Angel Rodriguez had done is nothing less than remarkable. He had lowered his body fat percentage from nearly 50 percent to just 11 percent in 30 weeks. Check out his before-and-after photos on the opposite page. He looks like an entirely different man—a younger man, a healthier man. Most important, he probably saved his own life by losing the weight.

The Gainesville Project

Rodriguez is one of more than 118 men and women who have achieved body-transforming, life-altering results, some recording up to a pound a day of fat loss, on average, over the course of just 30 to 50 days, on a revolutionary new diet and exercise program that I call the Body Fat Breakthrough. I tested this weight-loss system at one of the largest fitness facilities in the nation, 28,000-member Gainesville Health & Fitness in Florida in 2012.

It took 3 years to put this project together. Throughout this book, you'll learn more about the specifics. But for now, let me mention the following men:

→ **Joe Cirulli** is the owner Gainesville Health & Fitness. For 30 years, I've collaborated with Cirulli on numerous fat-loss and muscle-building projects and books involving test subjects from his club. Cirulli is a master at keeping his members motivated, active, and happy.

→ **Mats Thulin** is the inventor and owner of X-Force, the new negative-accentuated strength-training equipment that is manufactured in Stockholm, Sweden. When I tried X-Force for the first time in 2008, I knew I had to have a full line of X-Force available to me in Florida. Cirulli's Gainesville Health & Fitness was my choice for setting up the equipment. Thulin, Cirulli, and I developed a plan, and the equipment arrived in Gainesville in January 2012.

→ **Roger Schwab** is the owner of Main Line Health & Fitness in Philadelphia. Schwab is an experienced practitioner of strength training and bodybuilding, and I encouraged him to import a line of X-Force into his facility for testing and application. He agreed, and his equipment arrived in Philadelphia also in January 2012.

Cirulli, Thulin, Schwab, and others that you'll meet throughout this book worked with me tirelessly on the Gainesville project. The book you are holding in your hands and the program within it are the end result.

I have been a fitness researcher and writer for all my adult life. For 20 years, I was director of research at Nautilus Sports/Medical Industries, maker of the famed Nautilus fitness machines. I have a doctorate in exercise science and completed postdoctoral work in food and nutrition. I lecture on strength training and nutrition throughout the world and have been published in more than 75 research journals and magazines and have written 48 books.

The President's Council on Physical Fitness and Sports elected me as one of the top 10 Healthy American Fitness Leaders in the United States. I list my professional background not to show off but to give you the confidence that the advice and techniques I recommend for you in this book are safe, effective, and based on both scientific research and real-world examples from my experiment at Gainesville Health & Fitness.

BODY TRANSFORMATIONS

In this manual, you'll meet 35 of my most successful trainees through dramatic before-and-after photos and measurements. Before you read any further, I want you to thumb through the book and take a close look at those body-transformation photos. It's likely that someone in these pages has a body shape that is similar if not identical to yours. Just like that person, you can lose fat, build muscle, and reshape your body quickly . . . usually in 50 to 100 days and sometimes in as few as 30 days. Best of all, you'll start feeling and seeing it working within the first week. That's important, because the positive feedback that this program is designed to deliver quickly and often will help you stick to this new way of healthy living for life.

So get ready. Your journey to a leaner, stronger body is beginning.

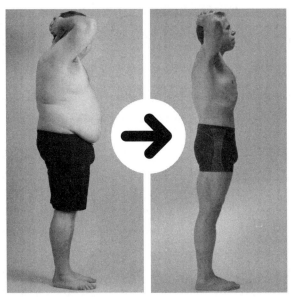

Rodriguez lost his belly and found muscle.

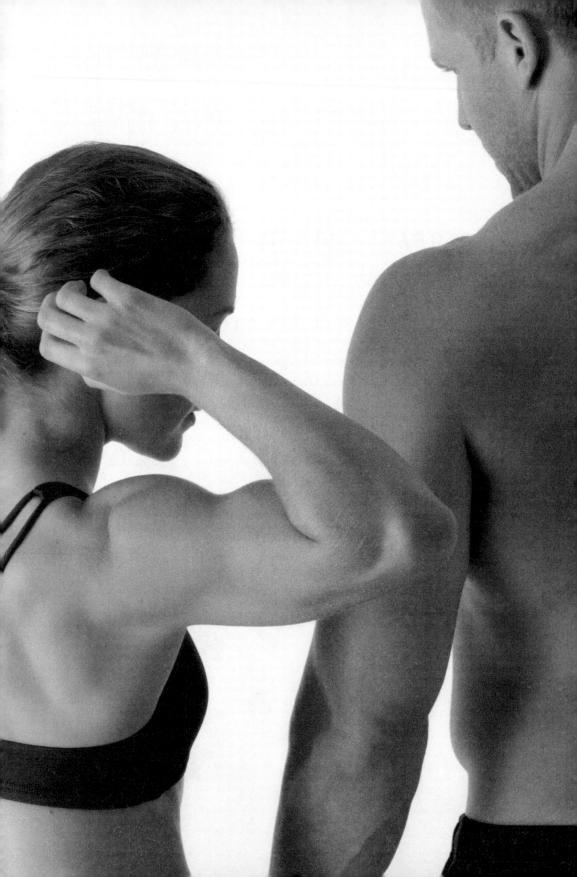

Proof Positive in Negative Training

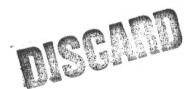

DAVID DOMASH

BEFORE & AFTER

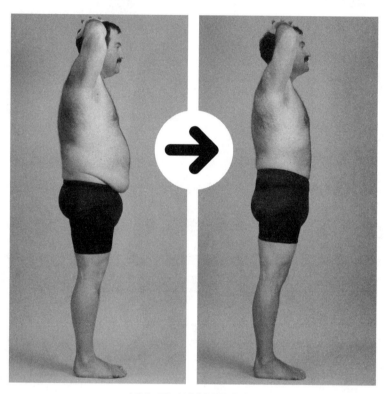

AGE 49, HEIGHT 5'8"

BEFORE BODY WEIGHT

208
POUNDS

AFTER BODY WEIGHT

174
POUNDS

AFTER 12 WEEKS

41.4
POUNDS OF FAT LOSS

9.75
INCHES OFF WAIST

7.4
POUNDS OF MUSCLE GAIN

CHAPTER 1

Fat Loss, Muscle Gain

How to drop up to 50 pounds of flab and 9 inches off your waist in 50 days!

IT'S safe to say that anyone who has dieted has been frustrated. Almost universally, when people attempt a diet program, they lose weight initially and sometimes quickly, only to have the weight come back. And often, they put on even more pounds after that initial tease of success.

Why does this happen? There's a simple reason, and it cuts to the core of what makes the Body Fat Breakthrough so different from every other weight-loss program: During your initial weight reduction on almost any other diet, you lost both fat and muscle. That's a key distinction, the muscle factor. You lose muscle while losing fat. Then, when you regain your lost weight—which almost always happens—you add back only fat because it's much, much easier to gain fat weight than it is to gain muscle weight. This is one reason why yo-yo dieting is such a bad idea. When you lose and regain weight repeatedly, you gradually get fatter and fatter because of the muscle loss that occurs each time you reduce your weight without doing proper exercise.

This is the dirty little secret of most popular diets: You will lose weight initially but gain back even more, and mostly fat, when you do not combine eating healthier (and consuming fewer calories) with muscle-maintaining exercise. Those programs that claim you can lose weight without doing a lick of exercise are lying to you. Sure, consuming more nutritious, less calorically dense foods is the key to weight loss, but your leaner body won't last unless you maintain it with muscle.

Your body has a "use it or lose it" mechanism for muscle. If you are sedentary, some of your muscle atrophies and is absorbed. Paradoxically, if your body senses famine (cutting calories), your body will hold on to its fat stores. These are survival mechanisms, and understanding them will help you see the light about how to achieve a leaner body for life.

The moral of the story is this: *Do not attempt to lose weight without training your muscles at the same time.* Prepare, plan, and persist . . . and get it right the first time. This book will show you exactly how to do it.

Understanding Important Concepts

Here are some fundamental ideas that you should familiarize yourself with before you embark on my Body Fat Breakthrough.

Body weight: Your body weight is simply what your entire body—which is composed of skin, hair, internal organs, bones, extracellular water, fat, and muscle—weighs. Body weight is measured on scales and is recorded in pounds or kilograms.

Weight loss: Comparing and subtracting two body weights taken over a certain period of time determines weight loss. Weight loss alone, because it includes at least seven different components, can be misleading. For example, it's possible over several days to become dehydrated and lose 5 to 10 pounds of body weight. Some diets seem to work wonders quickly because the pounds they shed come from your extracellular water and muscles—two components that you do not need to reduce. The vast majority of people need to lose fat specifically, more than they need to lose weight generally.

Fat loss: The average middle-aged American has layers of fat around the waist, hips, thighs, and torso and inside the abdomen. Not only is it ugly, but one type of fat—visceral fat that surrounds the internal organs—is dangerous, because it secretes unhealthy chemicals into our most important body parts. No wonder fat loss is the most sought-after goal in the entire fitness industry. If your goal is to lose fat, it's critical to know how much you have on your body right now so you can measure your progress. I measure a person's fat with the help of a Lange Skinfold Caliper. I record skin-fold measurements at three positions on the body and plug the total into a scientific formula that, according to age and gender, calculates the percentage of body fat. I multiply that by body weight to determine fat pounds. Subtracting a person's "after" fat pounds from his or her "before" fat pounds supplies me with a person's fat loss. And fat loss is a far superior body-composition guide than weight loss.

Muscle gain: Both men and women need more muscle. More muscle allows you to look better, perform better, and live longer stronger. Muscle also burns more calories, even at rest. You certainly don't need to decrease muscle from dieting or exercising—which is what happens in numerous programs. Almost everyone who progresses through my program loses significantly more fat pounds than weight pounds. That difference—fat loss minus weight loss—is the amount of muscle a person has built. The specific amount a trainee has built is what I call muscle gain.

The Lose Up to 30 Pounds in 30 Days concept: Fat loss and muscle gain are two benefits of my Breakthrough program. Equally important is to achieve both of them simultaneously. Doing so creates a synergistic action that allows some people to lose an incredible pound of fat a day for many consecutive days—indeed, weeks and months.

For example, my first and second research groups at Gainesville Health & Fitness involved 44 subjects (20 men and 24 women) and continued for 12 weeks. My most successful subject lost 80 pounds of fat over 80 days; 2 people lost 60 pounds in 60 days; 4 subjects lost 50 pounds in 50 days; 6 trainees lost 40 pounds in 40 days; and 7 participants lost 30 pounds in 30 days. In addition, my 3 top losers of fat in 50 days shrunk an average of 9.13 inches off their waistline circumference.

On the muscle-building side, each member of that initial 44-person test panel added, on average, 9.94 pounds of muscle—that's 9.94 pounds of muscle in 12 weeks, or 0.83 pound of muscle a week, which is an amazing group achievement.

If you are ever near Gainesville, Florida, you are invited to visit Gainesville Health & Fitness. It has earned a reputation throughout the United States for innovative fitness programs and high-quality service. If you pop in, keep your eyes open. You just may see some of the people featured in this book and even work out with them. They are wonderful people and eager to share what they've learned and experienced.

Make a Promise to Yourself

The before-and-after photographs in this book are proof positive of what you can achieve, too, if you make a strong commitment and join my Body Fat Breakthrough program.

It starts with commitment, a promise that you make to yourself to finally get into the best shape of your life. This is an important decision, because you are doing it not only for yourself but also for your family, the people who love you. And aren't they worth it?

Be aware that the Body Fat Breakthrough program, and losing up to a pound of fat per day, is not easy. It takes effort—but it's highly achievable. I mean, just look at all the people in this book who have done it. If they can do it, you can, too, by committing time and effort. Think about it: Have you ever done anything in your life that was meaningful, that you achieved without really trying? I seriously doubt it. Nothing worthwhile comes from luck or a secret, magic, effortless formula. Sit on a couch, watch TV, drink a delicious smoothie, lose weight. That's not realistic. If that's what you want, you won't find it here. Because it doesn't work.

What does work is regular effort and a disciplined approach. The Body Fat Breakthrough program is challenging and demanding, especially at first. But once you get the hang of what's required, it becomes *not easy* but what many participants call simple. There's a difference. *Easy* means little effort. *Simple* means it's not hard to understand or follow.

The Body Fat Breakthrough is simple because what you need to do to achieve success is outlined step-by-baby-step. That's right. You'll be introduced to 10 simple guidelines, which I call Fat Bombs. These are innovative techniques for losing fat. Add in some motivation and discipline on your part and you'll be able to reach your body-transformation goal by successfully applying my collection of tried-and-proven Fat Bombs to your daily life.

In the next chapter, I'll introduce you to one of the most efficient and effective Fat Bombs in the program. It's called negative-accentuated exercise. It's an amazing technique and the key reason why *breakthrough* is in the title of this book.

Soon you'll find out why.

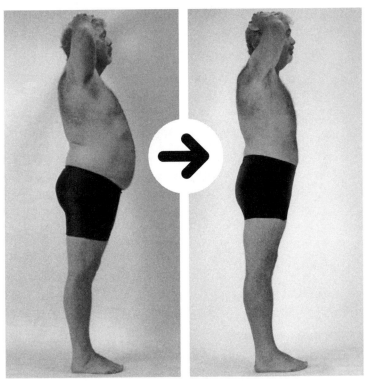

Storm Roberts was one of the participants who lost 30 pounds of fat in the first 30 days of the Breakthrough program. More details are presented on page 76. Roberts is a well-known morning show host on 98.5 KTK in the Gainesville area.

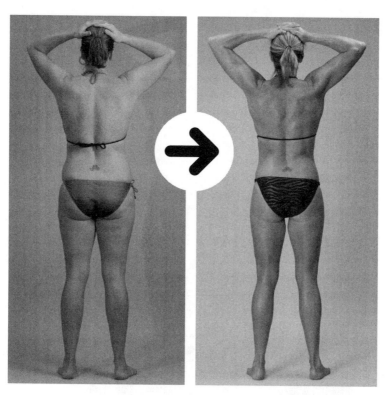

BODY FAT BREAKTHROUGH

ERIKA GREENE
BEFORE & AFTER

AGE 33, HEIGHT 5'6"

BEFORE BODY WEIGHT

146.5
POUNDS

AFTER BODY WEIGHT

133.75
POUNDS

AFTER 12 WEEKS

20.71
POUNDS OF FAT LOSS

5
INCHES OFF WAIST

7.96
POUNDS OF MUSCLE GAIN

CHAPTER 2

FAT BOMB #1:
Negative-Accentuated Strength Training

Try this breakthrough muscle-building, fat-torching exercise method

MORE muscle is your ticket to a better body. So even if you are a petite woman, don't be afraid of muscle-building exercises. You won't become muscle-bound; you will develop strength and well-toned, shapely muscles.

Take a close look at the after photos of Angel Rodriguez on page viii and Erika Greene on the opposite page. Notice the contours of Angel's and

Erika's upper arms and shoulders. How about Angel's forearms? Check out the muscularity in the middle of Erika's upper and lower back. Look at the lines in the thighs and calves. Angel's hamstrings, in his after side shot (see page xi), feature some of the best-developed back-thigh muscles that I've seen in my life.

Sure, both Angel and Erika lost significant body fat. But they also added pounds of muscle to their upper and lower bodies. Added muscle has given Angel and Erika tight, firm, and well-developed arms, shoulders, thighs, and calves. What's more, the extra muscle has increased their metabolic rates, so they burn more calories even at rest.

The Positive in the Negative

What's the best and most efficient way to add pounds of muscle to your body?

Until March 2012, my answer would have been high-intensity resistance exercise, which is a fancy way of saying weight lifting using increasingly more resistance or more repetitions and sets to all-out fatigue. In other words, really tough strength workouts. I've built a career researching this type of exercise. But now I've altered my thinking; my answer is more specific: negative-accentuated exercise.

That may sound technical, but it's really very simple. One way to explain negative-accentuated exercise is with a demonstration. Everybody knows what a pushup on the floor is like. You get on all fours, hands on the floor and directly under your shoulders, arms straight, on your toes with back flat from heels to head. Normally you lower your body and then push back up to the starting position. In a negative-accentuated pushup, however, what you're going to be doing is *only* the lowering portion—but you'll be performing it s-l-o-o-o-w-l-y.

"Heck, that should be easy," you might be thinking. "Just start at the top and drop to the bottom."

Not so fast. This version is anything but quick and easy. In fact, it's going to test your muscular power and force you to reexamine old habits. Your mission is to do the lowering phase of a pushup (from the elbows-straight position at the top to the elbows-bent position at the bottom) *as slowly as possible*. There is no pushing up. Your challenge involves only the lowering. You do the exercise once. Count as you go down. This rating scale will give you a sense of what I mean by slow:

→ 60-second lowering time: superior

→ 45-second lowering time: excellent

→ 30-second lowering time: good

→ 15- to 29-seconds lowering time: average

→ Below 15 seconds lowering time: an indication that your muscles need a lot of work

Try it right now. You'll need to outfit yourself in some tight-fitting clothes because you're going to be on the floor in a pushup situation. A blousy shirt and pants will mess you up, because the hanging material will make it difficult for you to judge your position on the floor.

LOWERING PUSHUP

Here are the directions to follow:

→ Get a friend who has a watch with a second hand to help with the counting. Your friend will be on one side of you in a low position where he or she can watch your elbows bend and count your lowering time.

→ Get on the floor. Place your hands shoulder-width apart, with your thumbs to the inside. Wear rubber-soled shoes and position your feet close together.

→ Assume the front-leaning-rest position, with your body off the floor and your arms fully extended but not locked.

→ Keep your legs, hips, midsection, and lower back straight. Do not allow any one of them to sag or arch. Do not drop your chin or extend your neck. The object is to lower your body, as a unit, very slowly—$\frac{1}{2}$ inch with each 5-second count—until your chest touches (but does not rest) on the floor and your elbows are fully bent.

→ Ready, start: Hold the top position with your arms straight for 5 seconds.

→ Bend your elbows slightly and lower your body just a little.

→ Hold firmly and lower another $\frac{1}{2}$ inch and then another $\frac{1}{2}$ inch. You should be approximately halfway down in 15 to 20 seconds.

→ Focus. Relax your face and neck, and don't hold your breath. In fact, breathe often.

→ Lower another $\frac{1}{2}$ inch and another $\frac{1}{2}$ inch. Keep your torso and hips in line. No sagging! Your goal is to be three-quarters down in 30 to 40 seconds. Your friend should be telling you the time in seconds: 25, 30, 35, 40.

→ Fight it when your chest is 1 inch from the floor. Hold for another 5 seconds, if possible.

→ Touch your chest to the floor and relax. The test is complete. What was your lowering time?

If you failed to get at least a 10-second lowering time, try the entire exercise again—but this time, perform it on your hands and knees. Doing the test from your hands and knees will be significantly easier than from your hands and toes. From the hands-and-knees position, you should still be able to feel the muscular contractions that occur in your triceps, deltoids, and pectorals.

MICROSCOPIC MUSCLE TEARS

If you were successful with the harder version for 30 to 60 seconds—even for as few as 20 seconds—you may have felt some "muscle stretching" across the front of your chest. Don't be alarmed.

Focused negative exercise, the kind that occurs when you first do the slow lowering part of a pushup, "can cause microscopic muscle tears, which ignite the protein-synthesis process," according to some of the best exercise physiologists in the world.

In 2009, Marc Roig, PhD, head of the Muscle Biophysics Laboratory at the University of British Columbia, and colleagues examined 66 studies reported within the past 50 years that compared negative-style resistance training with normal positive training. With precision, they applied meta-analyses to the data. In the most complete and meticulous literature review on the subject to date, Roig concluded that negative training was significantly more effective in increasing muscular size and strength than positive-style training.

The Difference between Positive and Negative Training

Here are a few clarifications on the words *negative* and *positive* as they relate to exercise, which may help you understand my point.

The word *positive* usually means "yes" or "good," and *negative* means "no" or "bad." But in the strength-training lexicon, *positive* refers to the raising or lifting part of the repetition. *Negative* means the lowering phase of a repetition.

In very simple terms, if you carefully observe a person's limbs in an activity or watch the weight stack during an exercise, then up is positive and down is negative.

The lowering phase of a pushup is a great example of negative training. Throughout this book, you will learn other exercises that accentuate the negative, or the lowering part of a movement.

Once again, scientific research shows—and my studies in Gainesville reinforce the science—that one of the best ways to build strength and muscle is to emphasize the lowering phase of many standard exercises.

A Tougher Challenge

In Gainesville, I focused on several ways to accentuate the negative, or make the lowering phase more intense, for each repetition. With almost any exercise performed with your body weight, free weights, or a weight-stack machine, you can make the negative phase harder by moving slower while lowering. Or you can lower for an extra half repetition.

For example, on the chest-press machine, try the following: Take 80 percent of the resistance that you normally use for pumping out 10 repetitions, up/down/up/down, fairly quickly, the typical way. Press the resistance quickly to the extended position. Then begin a very slow, 30-second lowering (similar to what you did on the negative pushup). Once you reach bottom, press the resistance in a slow, 30-second positive. Follow that with a final 30-second negative. You'll see; it won't be easy.

This style of negative-accentuated training involves two 30-second negatives and one 30-second positive. That's 1 1/2 repetitions in 90 seconds. This is an intense but productive method of training.

I'll demonstrate other ways to accentuate the negative, including several leading-edge versions, in Chapter 14. New exercise machines are being developed specifically for negative training. The best of these futuristic machines is X-Force, which I applied in Gainesville with outstanding results. More will be said about X-Force in the Appendix.

In the meantime, the flabby, out-of-shape situation in the United States needs some attention, which I'll address in the next chapter.

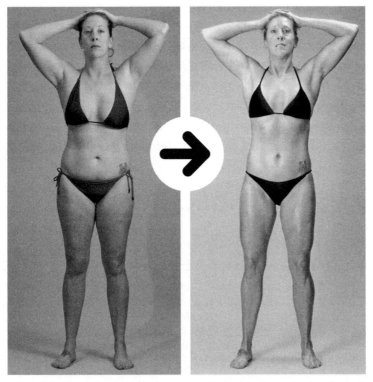

Erika Greene, featured on page 8 of this chapter, trained hard to firm and reshape her body. She trimmed 5 inches off her waist, 3.25 inches off her hips, and 3 inches off her thighs.

FAT BOMB #1

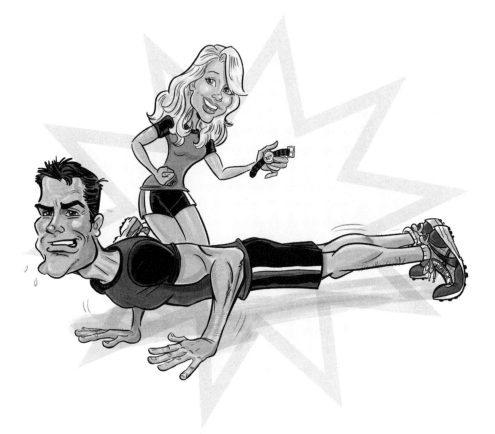

NEGATIVE-ACCENTUATED STRENGTH TRAINING

Emphasize the negative phase of each exercise by taking
significantly more time on the lowering, compared to the
lifting, of each repetition.

ASHLEY MEISNER
BEFORE & AFTER

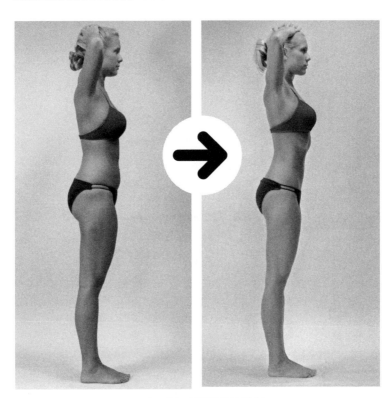

AGE 22, HEIGHT 5'8"

BEFORE BODY WEIGHT

143
POUNDS

AFTER BODY WEIGHT

127
POUNDS

AFTER 12 WEEKS

22.81
POUNDS OF FAT LOSS

6
INCHES OFF WAIST

6.81
POUNDS OF MUSCLE GAIN

Why We're So Fat

The hidden cause of a huge national health hazard

WE'VE all seen the statistics about how adults in the United States are fatter than they've ever been before (and kids, too). In the last year, if you've been to a public beach, an amusement park, a football game, a parade, a supermarket, or anywhere that crowds gather, you've seen people with excessive fat hanging from waists, upper backs, upper arms, necks, hips, and thighs. Perhaps you even see the same thing when you look in the mirror.

I could give you a lengthy lecture on the unhealthy eating habits that have contributed to the obesity of many Americans, but you've heard something similar before, numerous times. What I want to share with you is something you haven't heard, something you probably are not aware of, and something that you can improve quickly.

I'm talking about what's called disuse atrophy. Treating it will combat obesity effectively at the grassroots level.

Disuse Atrophy

There are about 700 named muscles in our bodies, and those muscles are divided into billions of tiny fibers. When a muscle grows, it increases the size of the involved fibers. The number of fibers doesn't increase, the size of them does, and this is what's known as hypertrophy.

The opposite of hypertrophy is atrophy. *Disuse atrophy* is when muscles shrink, or waste away, from lack of use. If a bodybuilder sat on the couch watching TV for a couple of months, his muscles would atrophy. Same goes for anyone—big muscles or not.

The late Gilbert Forbes, MD, of the Rochester School of Medicine did much of the basic research on disuse atrophy. I met Dr. Forbes in 1975; he helped me with a research project for Nautilus Sports/Medical Industries conducted at the U.S. Military Academy at West Point, New York. Dr. Forbes was very interested in the building of muscle mass.

At that time, Dr. Forbes was in the process of analyzing the body compositions of men and women he had monitored for several decades. His full report was published in the scientific journal *Human Biology* in 1976.

Basically, what he found was that average men and women between the ages of 20 and 50 who do not perform consistent heavy exercise lose half a pound of muscle per year. Scientists at the Nutrition, Exercise Physiology, and Sarcopenia Laboratory at Tufts University have reinforced Dr. Forbes's original 40-year-old research with the latest body-composition technology. It still stands: People typically lose half a pound of muscle per year of life. That 8 ounces of muscle per year translates into slightly more than $\frac{22}{100}$ ounce per day, which seems insignificant. But little by little, ounce by ounce, things add up. After a decade, it's 5 pounds. After 30 years, it's 15 pounds.

The next time you're at the supermarket, take a look at a 15-pound frozen turkey. That turkey is about the size of two footballs. Either of those examples is the approximate space in your body that 15 pounds of your muscle occupies.

A LITTLE HERE, A LITTLE THERE

Atrophy, however, is not selective. It happens throughout your body, from all of your major and minor muscles. Perhaps 2 pounds shrink from each thigh; another pound shrinks from each buttock, along with a couple of pounds from your back, chest, and shoulders and half a pound from each arm and each calf; and finally, the remaining several pounds shrink from around your lower back, midsection, and neck. Besides making you look and feel weaker, this disuse is likely to manifest itself in a physical ailment such as osteoarthritis, a degenerative disk, or even a heart attack. From there, it's usually a steady downward spiral. Muscle is that important to good health.

The shrinkage of muscle tissue from disuse involves metabolic breakdown of muscle into its constituent compounds, which are removed by the bloodstream. Atrophied muscle does not turn into fat. Muscle and fat are composed of different cells, and it's impossible to turn one into the other. Muscle cells that atrophy simply lose their fluids, become smaller and weaker, and lessen their ability to contract.

However, the fattening process affects the body in multiple ways. When the skin folds fill in, the girth and appearance of the limb can be similar to before, if not larger. The structure of the muscle also changes internally, with fat developing within the muscle. Fat hampers muscle function, reducing its ability to contract. When you lose muscle and what you have left becomes infused with fat, your ability to move and generate force is compromised.

Don't Ignore Your Muscles

Having bigger, stronger muscles may not be a panacea, but of all the factors over which you have some control, it is a critical one. Many of the aches and pains of old age can be averted. It is important that you understand the perils of ignoring muscle.

If you ever fractured a limb and spent several weeks in a cast, you have experienced a rapid atrophying of muscles from total immobility, along with accompanying pain in the joints. Without proper exercise, many of us place our entire bodies into a cast of sedentary living. The effects progress more slowly than what we experience with a fractured arm, but the results are just as damaging. Let's say you trip over a rock while walking. Your muscles' ability to react and contract, to move and support your skeleton so you can upright yourself, may mean the difference between catching your balance and slamming your head into the sidewalk. When you get into your eighties and nineties, muscle atrophy may keep you from rising out of a chair without someone's help.

With negative-accentuated training, you can put a stop to the regression and actually reverse the process. You can rebuild atrophied muscle and even build your muscles larger and stronger than they've ever been.

No, it won't be easy, especially if you are over 40. But it will be well worth it, as my Gainesville trainees will testify.

Creeping Obesity

While the typical man's or woman's body is losing a half pound of muscle each year between the ages of 20 and 50, his or her fat cells are thriving. The fat cell phenomenon progresses at three times the rate of muscle loss—only it's a gain, not a reduction. As far as your health and vitality are concerned, both situations are moving in the wrong direction.

So slowly are these dual physiological changes occurring that often it takes a decade or more to notice that something major has happened to your body.

The average adult over 3 decades gains 1.5 pounds of fat each year. That adds up to 15 pounds of extra fat per decade, or 45 pounds in 30 years. This slow accumulation of body fat is what nutritionists refer to as creeping obesity.

Actually, this creeping obesity is somewhat disguised by the shrinking of muscle mass that is going on at the same time. Let's say you lose 15 pounds of muscle through disuse atrophy over 30 years. Adding 45 pounds of fat through creeping obesity during that same time will appear on the scale as a weight gain of 30 pounds, not 45. In fact, the loss of muscle makes the situation worse. Here's why.

Your resting metabolic rate is the number of calories your body requires to function in a relaxed, resting state. Your brain and internal organs—such as your heart, lungs, liver, and kidneys—require a lot of energy. But it's your skeletal muscles, which make up from 30 to 50 percent of an average person's body weight, that use the most calories.

MORE MUSCLE MEANS LESS FAT

Add a pound of muscle to your body and your resting metabolic rate goes up 37.5 calories per day. Lose a pound through disuse atrophy and the opposite applies: Your rate is lowered by 37.5 calories per day.

Interestingly, a pound of fat also has a metabolic rate: approximately 2 calories per day. Muscle is 18.75 times as active metabolically as the same amount of fat.

You've probably noticed that it is more difficult to shed excess fat than it used to be. Long-term metabolic studies reveal that an average individual experiences a 0.5 percent reduction in metabolic rate each year between 20 and 50 years of age. The gradual loss of muscle mass is primarily responsible for this metabolic slowdown.

Certainly, controlling your dietary calories is an important aspect of combating creeping obesity—which I'll discuss in Part V. But equally important is rebuilding the size and strength you had at one time throughout your skeletal muscles.

Are you stuck with excessive fat cells and withered muscles? It's time to muscle your fat away with negative-accentuated exercise.

The next chapter shows why and how that is possible.

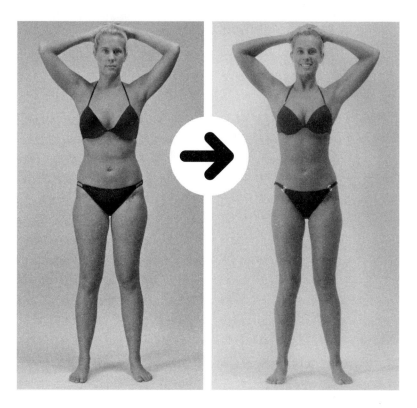

Ashley Meisner lost 6 inches from her waist and firmed up her bottom and thighs.

BOB SMITH
BEFORE & AFTER

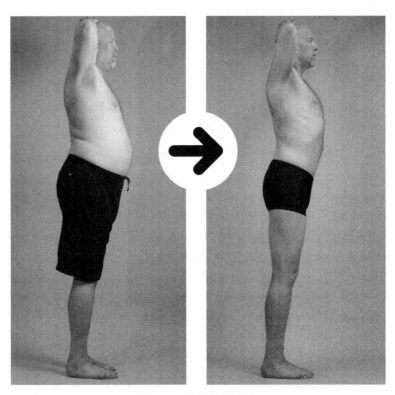

AGE 51, HEIGHT 6'7"

BEFORE BODY WEIGHT

302
POUNDS

AFTER BODY WEIGHT

232
POUNDS

AFTER 18 WEEKS

94
POUNDS OF FAT LOSS

11.5
INCHES OFF WAIST

24
POUNDS OF MUSCLE GAIN

Building Muscle and Losing Fat

Learn the secret formula for remarkable results

ON February 6, 2012, I began my first negative-accentuated exercising and eating study at Gainesville Health & Fitness in Gainesville, Florida. The subjects were 40 women and 25 men, each of whom needed to lose 20 or more pounds of fat.

The two heaviest men in the group were Jim Deason, at 6 feet tall and a starting body weight of 346 pounds, and Bob Smith (shown on opposite page), at 6 feet 7 inches tall and a body weight of 302 pounds. Both of the men were intense trainees on the negative-accentuated routines, and each man's body weight was dropping at the rate of 5 pounds per week—which was what I expected for men who weighed 300 pounds.

During studies like this, I typically have two or three group meetings, usually on Sunday afternoons. During these meetings, I discuss progress, answer questions, and review what's ahead for the next week. It was the close of the March 17 meeting, and I had just reviewed all the guidelines for taking everyone's after measurements and photographs, which was set for the next 2 days. It was imperative that each participant arrive at the fitness center in the correct bathing suit at the appropriate time, so my assistants were busy double-checking the schedules for both days.

Jim Deason approached me with a concerned look on his face. He was a video producer, and he had to be in Jacksonville for the next 4 days, so he couldn't attend the photo session. But he'd brought his bathing suit, just in case I could take some of his measurements then.

Since Jim was one of my best trainees, I didn't want to remove him from the study, nor did I want to delay his measurements for another week, so I agreed to meet him in the dressing room in 5 minutes to get his skin-fold and body-weight numbers.

In the dressing room, I hastily removed my skin-fold caliper from its case and told Jim to stand tall with his right hand on his right hip. Quickly, I took several skin-fold measurements on Jim's chest, abdomen, and thigh—and wrote them down on a small piece of paper. Then I hustled him over to the medical scales for an official weigh-in.

I totaled the caliper numbers, looked at a chart, and recorded Jim's percentage of body fat. Then I had to locate his before measurement sheet from a folder at the bottom of my bag. Next I had to subtract his after body weight from his before body weight and compare that number with Jim's total fat pounds lost.

A participant's fat loss is a straightforward calculation. You simply subtract the after number of fat pounds from the before number. Muscle gain is achieved in an indirect manner. What I do is subtract weight loss from fat loss. Ninety-five percent of the time, fat loss is greater than weight loss. Thus, the difference between those two numbers is the amount of muscle a trainee has gained.

I did some fast calculations on Jim's numbers, and I was shocked. Jim had gained 14.5 pounds of muscle in 6 weeks, the most muscle gained of any subject I'd ever worked with in any one of my fat-loss studies. That's significant, since over the past 40 years, I've done more than 30 studies that involved more than 1,000 subjects. Furthermore, Jim's fat loss was 42.5 pounds, which was amazing.

Early the next morning, I was still thinking about Jim Deason and his 14.5-pound muscle gain. The first person who came in for the day's measurements and photos was big Bob Smith. With care, I recorded his skin-fold measurements. Then I took them again and even a third time.

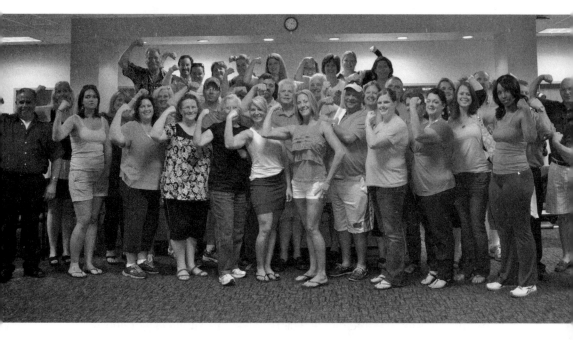

Members of my Group 1 study pose after completing 6 weeks of the Breakthrough program. Collectively, that extra muscle helped them lose more than 1,177 pounds of fat.

I repeated them twice because of my experience with Jim Deason the night before. But even then, I could hardly believe what Bob's numbers revealed: a gain of exactly 20 pounds of muscle. I knew from having pushed Bob through about half of his workouts that he was the hardest working of our participants, but still, his results blew me away. Bob Smith's 20 pounds of muscle gain beat Jim Deason's 12-hour-old record of 14.5 pounds. And Bob lost 54 pounds of fat in 6 weeks, which was also an all-time fat-loss record for people I have worked with over the past 40 years.

Wow! What was going on?

What was the probability that the first two participants for my after measurements would break my 2-decades-old record of 12.5 pounds of muscle gain in 6 weeks?

Interestingly, by the end of the second day of measurements, I had recorded seven participants who had built at least 10 pounds of muscle—and two of them were women.

My men's negative-accentuated group and women's negative-accentuated group, compared with all my previous groups, had established new records in average muscle gain—not by a little but by a lot.

My men's and women's groups also set records for fat-loss averages.

However, the real headliners were Bob Smith and Jim Deason. They finished in the number one and number two positions in both the muscle-gain and fat-loss categories. I've never had two men build so much muscle and lose so much fat simultaneously in only 6 weeks.

For 40 years, I've known that building muscle and losing fat together, on a lower-calorie diet, is possible. I've worked with hundreds of people who have experienced it. I've personally experienced it. And I've written a dozen books that explain how to do it. But the results were always moderate at best—nothing like those achieved by Bob Smith and Jim Deason.

The Secret Formula

I knew on the night of March 19, 2012, that I was close to a potential discovery of real value. I knew that it had to do with the way the subjects were performing their negative-accentuated exercise, with no resting between repetitions.

I just needed most of the subjects to continue for another 6 weeks, so I could collect more data. I was fortunate—most of the participants did continue. I'll share that data and the complete results in Chapter 6.

In the meantime, I've had a chance to analyze some of the reasons why building muscle has such a tremendous influence on losing fat. It comes down to the power of hormones.

A hormone is a chemical messenger released by a gland, or a cell, in one part of the body and delivers messages that affect cells in other parts of the organism. Hormones work slowly and affect many different processes, including:

- *growth and development*
- *metabolism*
- *mood*
- *sexual function*
- *reproduction*

Endocrine glands, which are special groups of cells, make hormones. The major endocrine glands are the pituitary, pineal, thymus, thyroid, adrenal, and pancreas. In addition, men produce hormones in their testes and women produce them in their ovaries.

Hormones are powerful. It takes only a tiny amount to cause big changes in cells or even your whole body.

I've been interested in bodybuilding for more than 50 years, so I'm well aware of the legal and illegal ways to activate, or supplement, the various hormones that play a role in muscle development. I have read thousands of books and articles on the subject.

I have a 24-year-old daughter, Sarah, who has entered a bodybuilding contest. And I have a son, Tyler, 11, whom I've been training since he was 3. I've watched them both—and two more children of mine as well—eat, exercise, rest, sleep, and grow. Plus, I have a strong, muscular wife, who is also interested in hard training. My point is that I'm not interested in bodybuilding for the vanity aspect; rather, I want muscle building to be a beneficial and healthy activity for my family, and I want it to be beneficial and healthy for you, too.

Hormones and Muscle Building

When it comes to muscle development, the most widely researched hormones are testosterone, insulin-like growth factor (IGF-1), and growth hormone (GH). Plus, there's a related hormone called interleukin 6 (IL-6), which comes from the muscle itself. Here's what basic research shows.

Testosterone: This hormone promotes muscle growth in three ways. First, it directly improves protein synthesis and inhibits protein breakdown. Second, it activates satellite cells, which supplement the muscle-building process. Third, it can indirectly contribute to protein buildup by stimulating other hormones involved in anabolism, or the building up of tissue.

In males, testosterone is produced mostly in the testes. Females produce only a small fraction of the testosterone that males do, which is the main reason most women find it difficult to develop muscle bulk.

Insulin-like growth factor: Several types of IGF-1 have been isolated. Two of them—a systemic version that is released by the liver and a muscle-specific form called mechano-growth factor (MGF) that is activated by muscle contraction—appear to be instrumental in muscle adaptation. Currently, MGF is thought to be the more important of the two forms. MGF is especially sensitive to muscle stretching, tearing, and soreness. Under those conditions, MGF may kick-start the entire muscular-growth process.

Growth hormone: Interestingly, most of the anabolic effects of GH are probably related to its synergistic relationship with IGF-1. GH, in fact, seems to have a greater effect on reducing body fat than on building muscle. Evidently, GH promotes the use of fat as fuel.

Interleukin 6: Muscular contraction, especially the negative action, stimulates interleukin-6 and its receptor, IL-6Ra, which are chemical messengers that help with the repair and overcompensation of muscle damage and inflammation. IL-6 also helps in the breakdown of fat stored in fat cells.

Besides prototypical IL-6, there's recent discovery of interleukin 15 (IL-15). IL-15 has been labeled a primary example of muscle-fat cross talk. Under the right conditions, it helps synergize the building of muscle and the loss of fat.

Educated Thoughts

People have a lot of questions and concerns about hormones. My Gainesville participants had many, and I'm sure you do, too. Let me share what I know by answering some frequently asked questions. Note: There are no definitive answers to these questions. The mechanisms of muscle growth are very complex, and many interactions are required.

The best I can do is supply you with my educated thoughts, based on the studies I've read, combined with the familiarity of training 145 subjects in Gainesville, plus my more than 50 years of related experience.

Furthermore, I'm assuming that readers of this book have natural levels of testosterone that respond in a normal manner, so I will not include testosterone in the discussion below.

Q: *What is it about negative-accentuated exercise that causes so much muscular-growth stimulation?*

A: *With the negative-accentuated style, you are making a 40 to 50 percent greater "inroad" into your starting level of strength, compared with the regular style of training. Inroad, in simple terms, is stress, the amount of activation of muscle fibers that comes from a repetition or complete set of an exercise.*

I believe this deeper inroad stimulates five key hormones—MGF, IL-6, IL-15, IGF-1, and GH—to start pulsating into the bloodstream and trigger physiological changes. Over the next 72 to 120 hours, with the right conditions, muscular growth occurs.

Q: Why does negative exercise make me so tired?

A: *Feeling tired comes from a combination of deeper inroad, hormonal stimulations, and your body telling you that it must get more rest, recovery, and sleep—sleep that's deeper than normal. Speaking of deeper sleep, have you ever noticed how children— especially when they are having growth spurts—tend to sleep deeper and longer? Sometimes it seems as though a loud freight train running by their beds couldn't wake them up. I believe that IGF-1 and GH are contributing factors in both cases.*

Q: How does negative-accentuated exercise contribute to fat loss?

A: *Muscular growth, especially if the person is adhering to a reduced-calorie eating plan, pulls calories from fat cells. IL-15 and GH, once they circulate, oxidize fat-cell content at a faster-than-normal rate.*

Q: Why does negative-accentuated exercise make me so hungry?

A: *Spiking your appetite is one of your body's first responses to trying to build muscle. Your body would rather get its muscle-building calories from food, as opposed to pulling them from the fat-storage cells.*

Q: What can I do to recover faster from negative-accentuated exercise?

A: *Your negative-accentuated recovery ability improves if you consume a carbohydrate-rich diet. That's one reason my fat-loss eating plan is so different from the popular high-protein diets. It's composed of 50 percent carbohydrates.*

It may be that the negative-accentuated deeper inroad, combined with just the right amount of carbohydrates, decreases insulin responsiveness in fat cells and they shrink. Apparently, as insulin sensitivity in muscle increases, nutrients are guided into muscle cells, and they expand.

Remember: Build muscle to lose fat. That's a big part of the success of the Body Fat Breakthrough program.

HERB JONES
BEFORE & AFTER

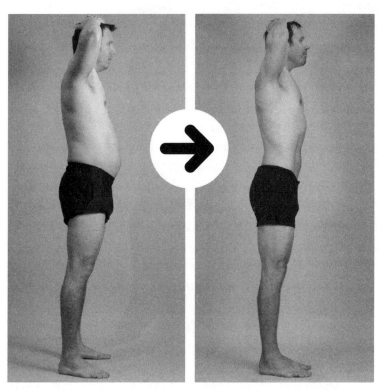

AGE 42, HEIGHT 6'0"

BEFORE BODY WEIGHT

212
POUNDS

AFTER BODY WEIGHT

188
POUNDS

AFTER 12 WEEKS

35.96
POUNDS OF FAT LOSS

7.375
INCHES OFF WAIST

11.96
POUNDS OF MUSCLE GAIN

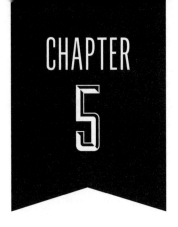

CHAPTER 5

FAT BOMB #2:
A Cold Burn

Try this newly discovered recovery method

PICTURE THIS: a 500-pound male black bear asleep in a cave in the mountains. This bear has a heavy coat of fur and, underneath, a thick layer of fat that helps him maintain his body temperature for 3 months through the winter. But as spring arrives and the temperatures rise, he awakes and lumbers outside the cave.

Question: How does a 500-pound, well-insulated bear move around actively, find food, and protect himself without overheating?

For years, that was a question that bugged H. Craig Heller, PhD, and Dennis Grahn, PhD, biologists at Stanford University. Heller and Grahn finally discovered that bears and, in fact, nearly all mammals have built-in radiators: hairless areas of the body with networks of veins close to the surface of the skin that help dissipate heat when the time is right.

Dogs have them in their tongues; elephants, in their ears; and rats, in their tails. When you examine a thermal scan of a bear, the animal is almost indistinguishable from its background, except . . . the pads of its feet and the tip of its nose look as though they are on fire. Networks of veins in these areas have highly variable bloodflow, ranging from almost none in cold weather to 60 percent of cardiac output in hot weather or during vigorous activity. They help our woolly bear keep from overheating in spring and summer.

In humans, the veins are prevalent in several places: the face, the feet, and—the most prominent radiator structures—the palms of the hands. Knowing how these temperature regulators work has practical applications in medicine and physical therapy and, as you'll soon find out, in the Body Fat Breakthrough program.

Muscles and Heat Sensitivity

In experiments, biologists Heller and Grahn devised a rigid plastic glove to place on one hand. Attached to the mitt was a hose that created a slight vacuum. Then the vacuum circulated cold water through the glove. As a result, the network of veins throughout the hand cooled rapidly.

At first, Heller and Grahn tried using the glove during postsurgery situations to alter body temperature, which proved very effective in patients recovering from anesthesia. Later, an athletic colleague applied the glove to cool his hand between sets of chinups on a horizontal bar. The glove seemed to erase muscle fatigue between sets. The researchers then applied the cooling glove to other exercises, such as the bench press with a barbell, running, and cycling. In all individuals, rates of muscle gain in recovery were significant, without any evidence of damage to the body from overwork.

But how does body temperature relate to muscle fatigue? Only recently did we learn the answer.

In 2009, researchers discovered that muscle pyruvate kinase, an enzyme that muscles need to generate chemical energy, is extremely sensitive to temperature. At normal body temperature, the enzyme functions well. But as temperatures rise, the enzyme begins to deform. At a muscle temperature of

104°F, there's no enzyme activity. It shuts down completely. As more stress is placed on a muscle fiber, it registers more internal heat. If the process continues for too long, the fiber will self-destruct. But if the ability to contract stops before the critical temperature is reached, an individual can no longer continue the movement. Thus, muscle pyruvate kinase supplies a crucial self-regulation system for the muscle by preventing contraction.

According to Heller and Grahn, your muscle fibers are saying that you can't work intensely anymore, because if you do, you're going to cook from the inside out and die! But when you cool the muscle fibers, you return the enzyme to the active state by resetting the muscle's state of fatigue.

You might be thinking that instead of using the glove, why not just stick your hand in a bucket of cold water or ice?

That doesn't work well because doing so will certainly cool your hand, but it will also cause the blood vessels to shut down so the cooled blood is not transported to your core. Getting most of your body into a tub of cold water, however, would circulate blood to your core.

Cold Experiences

It was the first week of September 2012 when I read the news from Stanford University about black bears, the networks of surface veins that radiate heat, and the vacuum cold glove. That wasn't the first time, however, I'd heard about the physiological benefits of getting cold.

In 1972, at the Olympic Games in Munich, Germany, I heard discussions about Olympic wrestlers from Middle Eastern countries sleeping in cold environments, with no clothes nor covers, to lose a couple of extra pounds of fat before their official weigh-ins. These wrestlers said that an almost-shivering state required three times as many calories, compared with sweating, to keep the body regulated. Ten years later, I read about a study in which subjects submerged themselves chin deep in cold water and burned more calories than normal, in an attempt to lose fat faster. Those two bits of information prompted me in 1985 to recommend to my fat-loss research subjects the concept of keeping cool, as opposed to sweating, to burn more calories each day.

In 2008, Joe Cirulli, the owner of Gainesville Health & Fitness and a fitness buff, told me about his first experience of submerging himself in his club's new cold plunge. Joe had heard good reports from a few fitness centers that had installed cold-plunge areas in their clubs to help clients lose weight. So during his next club expansion, he put in a 10-feet-square area in the back, near his swimming pool, and specifically outfitted it with regulators to keep the water at a chilly 52°F. Soon many of his members loved taking a brief cold plunge after a hard workout. Most reported that the cold water seemed to eliminate many of their lower-body aches and pains. But Joe had not tried the cold water, and the area had been in operation for 3 months.

So he developed a plan.

One of Joe's most grueling workouts involved going inside the University of Florida's football stadium and running up and down the stairs next to the tiered rows of seats. There were 80 rows of seats on the side that Joe ran. And and he usually went up and down five times. That always made his hips, thighs, and calves so sore that for almost a week, he had trouble sitting down.

His plan was to repeat the above routine and afterward, add the cold plunge.

But on the stadium-run day, he decided to really push himself, so he ran up and down the steps seven times. By the time he made it back to GHF and the cold plunge, he could barely walk.

As he eased into the 52°F water, a couple of friendly members joined him and engaged him in conversation. Before he knew it, 20 minutes had elapsed. By that time his teeth were chattering, so Joe staggered out, took a hot shower, and drove home—where, he said, he had to put on a heavy coat, eat two bowls of hot soup, and drink a couple of cups of hot tea, just to stop his shivering.

But guess what? When Joe got out of bed the next morning, he felt no soreness. Not the next day, either, nor the day after. *None.* Cold also minimizes the microtrauma in the muscle fibers following a workout. Subsequently, as the chilled tissue warms, the increased bloodflow speeds circulation—which, in turn, makes the recovery process more efficient. Reducing the inflammatory process seems to reduce the residual soreness associated with intense exercise, especially negative versions.

Joe's stadium story sealed the deal for me. Beginning in February 2012, I decided to encourage all my fat-loss groups in Gainesville to take a cold plunge for 5 to 10 minutes after their negative-accentuated workouts. Approximately half of the first group of 55 subjects used the cold plunge at least once a week. The guy who was the most consistent cold plunger was Herb

Jones. And it showed. Herb lost 35.96 pounds of fat and built 11.96 pounds of muscle. He reduced his body fat to 8.5 percent, which was the lowest level of any participant.

The cold-plunge practice continued nicely from February through August. Then I read about the black bears and the Stanford research. Quickly, I had two ideas that could improve the results of the cold plunge at GHF.

First, all our trainees had been getting into the cold plunge at navel-deep level. After several minutes, they eased their torsos slightly deeper and endured for another 7 or 8 minutes. But the entire time was made more tolerable by keeping their hands and forearms completely above the water. But after reading about the Stanford research, I knew the effect on the overall recovery, as well as the calorie burn, would be more significant with the hands and forearms under the water.

Second, many of our trainees, before getting into the plunge, would put on a pair of rubberized shoe socks to keep their feet a little warmer. I realized that these warming shoes or socks prevented some of the radiant effects of feet and the cold water. So no more rubberized shoe socks.

Plunge Pointers

Personally, I've used the cold plunge multiple times, always with good results. Here are some additional guidelines to practice if you take the plunge:

→ Be conservative with the water temperature. Most rehabilitation specialists recommend a water temperature of 54° to 60°F. GHF keeps their cold plunge at 52° to 54°F.

→ Don't assume that colder is better. Spending time in water colder than 52°F can be dangerous. On the other hand, 60° to 75°F water can still be beneficial.

→ Keep your feet and hands underwater.

→ Stay in the cold plunge for 5 minutes initially. Gradually work up to 7 to 8 minutes. Do not exceed 10 minutes.

→ Ease out of the cold plunge and wait 5 minutes before you shower.

ALTERNATIVES

If you don't have access to a cold plunge, I don't expect you to jump in a lake. There are other ways to reap similar benefits. Try these:

Take a cold shower. Ease into a hot shower and let the hot water hit your entire body for 2 minutes. Step out of the hot water and apply shampoo to your hair. Lather up your head. Switch the water to pure cold and rinse your head and face alone. Rotate and back quickly into the cold water. Focus the spray on your lower neck and upper back. Maintain this position for 1 to 3 minutes. As you acclimatize, soap the rest of your body. Turn around and rinse normally. Exit the shower, shivering as you go, and towel yourself dry.

Put an ice pack on your neck. Icing down your neck may activate what's known as brown fat, a special adipose tissue fat that helps get rid of excess calories as heat.

I read about the calorie-burning effects of brown fat more than 30 years ago. Brown fat is brownish in color and appears to be derived from the same stem cells as muscle tissue.

Black bears have a lot of brown fat over their necks and shoulders, which also tends to be where humans store it in much smaller amounts. Interestingly, cold temperatures cause brown fat to burn regular subcutaneous fat at a higher rate than normal—in both black bears and humans.

That's why for accelerated fat loss, you can try placing a U-shaped ice pack around the back of your neck and upper trapezius for approximately 30 minutes in the evening, three times per week. Several of my participants have tried this technique, and they seem pleased with the overall results.

FAT BOMB #2

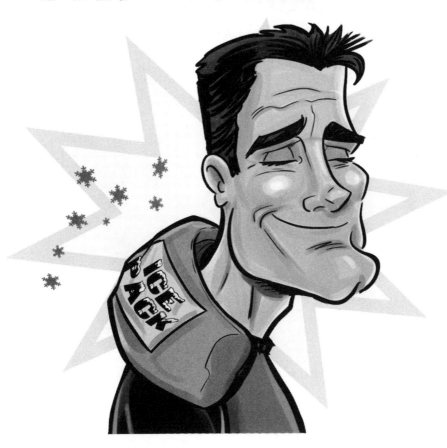

HOW ABOUT A COLD ONE?

Not a cold brew – but a cold pack around the back of your
neck after an intense workout.

MELISSA NORMAN

BEFORE & AFTER

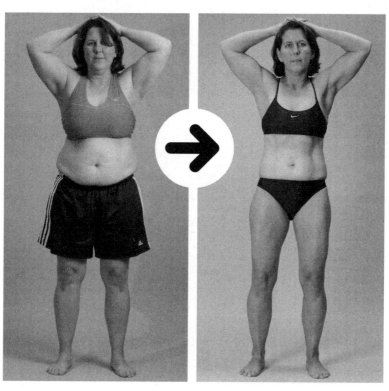

AGE 42, HEIGHT 5'2"

BEFORE BODY WEIGHT

173
POUNDS

AFTER BODY WEIGHT

129.4
POUNDS

AFTER 24 WEEKS

52.2
POUNDS OF FAT LOSS

12.625
INCHES OFF WAIST

8.6
POUNDS OF MUSCLE GAIN

CHAPTER

6

A Breakthrough in Gainesville

Inspiring losses and gains to get you motivated

ON January 29, 2012, I spoke to a gathering of approximately 150 Gainesville Health & Fitness members, each of whom needed to lose 20 or more pounds of fat. Forty women and 25 men were selected for my first group. Each person was weighed, measured, and photographed in a bathing suit.

All the subjects started my 6-week fat-loss plan on February 6, 2012. The women consumed approximately 1,300 calories a day, and the men ate approximately 1,500 calories a day. In addition, the participants were instructed to drink at least 1 gallon of cold water daily.

All participants were trained on one set of four or five negative-accentuated exercises twice a week at the fitness center. Six instructors, my assistant, and I supervised the training. The subjects were divided into five subgroups of 10 to 12 trainees, with each subgroup exercising at a scheduled time. Halfway through the study, we reduced the frequency from twice a week to once a week and increased the number of exercises from five to eight.

My goal for Group 1: to motivate and instruct each participant to apply the negative-accentuated exercise properly and adhere to the reduced-calorie eating plan strictly. Also, I wanted to compare the results of Group 1 to the best fat-loss and muscle-gain averages described in my book *A Flat Stomach ASAP*.

The Group 1 posttesting took place on March 19 and 20, 2012. Ten participants dropped out, so the data below included 34 women and 21 men.

Group 1: Averages after 6 Weeks

2012 NEGATIVE-ACCENTUATED GROUP 1

MEN (n = 21)

Age: 48.2 years

Height: 70.83 inches

Starting body weight:
248.25 pounds

Fat loss: 29.45* pounds

Muscle gain: 8.83* pounds

*27% more fat loss
*120% more muscle gain

WOMEN (n = 34)

Age: 42.71 years

Height: 65.59 inches

Starting body weight:
187.53 pounds

Fat loss: 16.85* pounds

Muscle gain: 5.1* pounds

*13% more fat loss
*46% more muscle gain

1998 ASAP GROUP

MEN (n = 41)

Age: 36.3 years

Height: 70.5 inches

Starting body weight:
208.3 pounds

Fat loss: 23.1 pounds

Muscle gain: 4 pounds

WOMEN (n = 109)

Age: 37.4 years

Height: 64 inches

Starting body weight:
156.5 pounds

Fat loss: 14.94 pounds

Muscle gain: 3.5 pounds

The fat-loss and muscle-gain averages over 6 weeks for the Negative-Accentuated Group were impressive. In fact, Group 1 set many new records. The Negative-Accentuated Group averaged a fat loss of 29.45 pounds, which was 27 percent more fat loss than the previous best, 23.1 pounds. The average muscle gain for the Negative-Accentuated Group was 8.83 pounds per man, while the old record from 1998 was 4 pounds—a 120 percent improvement.

The women in the Negative-Accentuated Group registered a 13 percent average increase in fat loss—16.85 pounds, compared with 14.94 pounds. In muscle gain, the women in the Negative Group averaged 5.1 pounds, compared with the ASAP Group average of 3.5 pounds—a noteworthy 46 percent improvement.

Simple division showed that the average man lost 0.7 pound of fat each day and 4.91 pounds each week. The average woman lost 0.4 pound of fat each day and 2.81 pounds each week. In terms of muscle gain, the average man built 1.47 pounds of muscle each week, and the average woman gained 0.85 pound each week. Those average fat-loss and muscle-gain numbers are beyond extraordinary, far and away better than any other group I've ever organized and directed. I have been conducting similar studies since 1966, and to the best of my knowledge, these results are unparalleled; no other researcher has ever recorded outcomes even close to these.

Now, that is a real breakthrough.

Group 2: Averages after 12 Weeks

Forty-five of 55 participants from the first 6 weeks signed up and continued for another 6 weeks. The second 6-week subjects, called Group 2, started on March 26, 2012, and finished on May 7, 2012. There was only one dropout.

The major difference between the negative-accentuated schedules for Group 1 and Group 2 was that Group 2 trained only once a week. The participants performed one set of eight negative-accentuated exercises under supervision for 6 consecutive weeks. Below are the averages for the men and the women.

MEN (n = 20)	WOMEN (n = 24)
Age: 50.8 years	**Age:** 42.04 years
Height: 70.66 inches	**Height:** 65.29 inches
Starting body weight: 248.88 pounds	**Starting body weight:** 197.08 pounds
Fat loss: 42.29 pounds	**Fat loss:** 27.47 pounds
Muscle gain: 13.38 pounds	**Muscle gain:** 7.21 pounds

Once again, the results were exceptional. This group realized fat-loss and muscle-gain averages for both men and women significantly above any other groups that I've worked with.

Groups 3 through 8

Group 3 involved 15 men and 12 women, and all of them were interested in bodybuilding. None of them wanted to lose fat. They trained once a week on a negative-accentuated routine for 6 weeks. No additional exercise of any kind was allowed. Their dietary calories were not reduced. In fact, they were encouraged to eat a few hundred more calories than normal each day.

For the remainder of 2012, June through mid-December, five smaller groups of subjects embarked on supervised negative-accentuated programs for 6 weeks. Fifty-three subjects, 31 women and 22 men, finished the course. And in each of the five groups, there were always 5 to 10 participants who

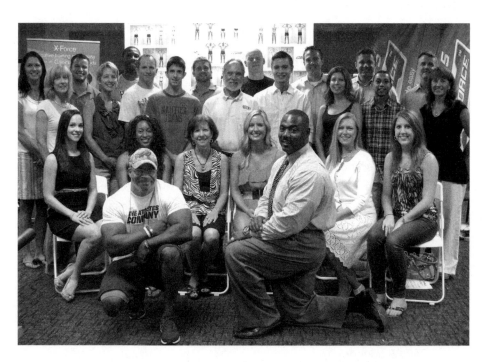

Group 3 was composed of individuals who were primarily interested in building muscle. In 6 weeks, they added 192 pounds of muscle to their bodies.

were repeats from an earlier group. A grand total of 145 subjects progressed through one or more of my 6-week courses in 2012. Of that total, 118 subjects (77 women and 41 men) were chosen for fat loss.

My test panels were filled with a broad spectrum of people of all ages interested in improving their bodies and their health. There were several doctors, lawyers, homemakers, and college students. There was an accountant, a pastor, a nurse, a mother of four, a grocer, a firefighter, a policeman, an insurance executive, and a chef. The 145 subjects were a mixture of Americans, but almost everyone was overfat and out of shape with their personal reasons for getting involved and personal demons to combat.

As I said in Chapter 1, the Body Fat Breakthrough program is challenging and demanding. Why? Because losing fat and building muscle are challenging and demanding. Both take a lot of hard work.

But the information and illustrations contained within this book will make it seem as though my staff and I are on hand to personally supervise you as you join the other 145 participants.

SIMPLE, STRAIGHTFORWARD . . . AND QUICK!

Thumb through this book one more time and examine the before-and-after photos. There's probably someone in the group that resembles you. Read how long it took him or her to get significant results. You can do the same.

Now turn to page 305. You'll see all 10 Breakthrough guidelines on one page. These are what I call my Fat Bombs. Taken as a group, they may seem overly complex. *Stop.* What you've done to yourself over the last several years, or several decades, is what got you into a complex condition. So, yes, it may seem complex and complicated. But, facing reality head-on and tackling each Fat Bomb one at a time, as recommended in this book, the process becomes *not easy* but simple. I promise. You can use the Fat Bombs to change your life. Give them a try and you'll see how effective they are. With your dedicated application, the results will be quick.

Close your eyes and picture the leaner, stronger body you'll have in just 6 weeks.

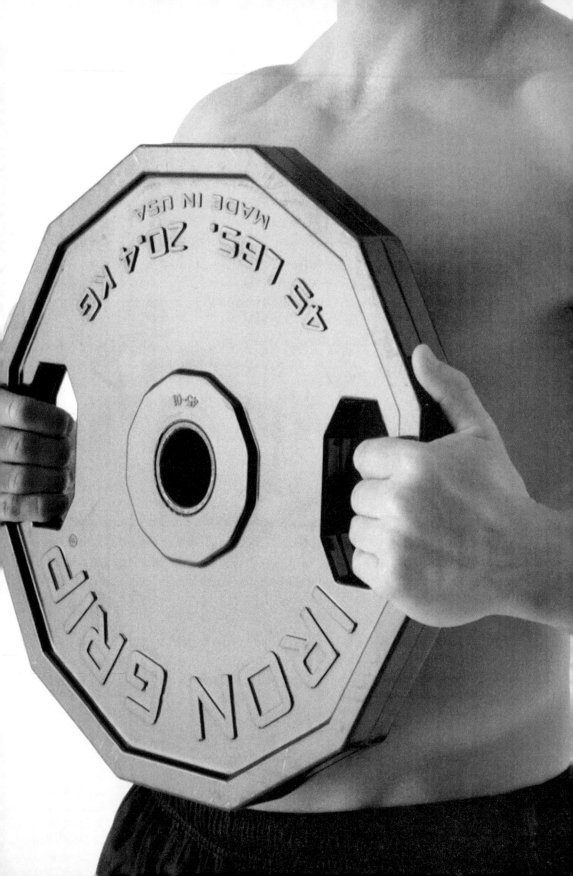

PART

II

The Roots of the Body Fat Breakthrough

CHAPTER 7

How Much Can You *Lower*?

Old-school practices that work wonders today

IN Part II I'll share a bit of history about my special interest in muscle building and I'll introduce some of the men who've influenced me throughout this journey.

If you want to get started on the 6-week Body Fat Breakthrough plan sooner, like tomorrow, rather than later, go right into the meat of the program, which begins in Part VI.

From my tenure of 20 years as director of research for Nautilus Sports/Medical Industries, I had rich experiences working with various athletes and nonathletes, some of which I recorded in my books:

- ***The Nautilus Diet* (1987)**
- ***32 Days to a 32-Inch Waist* (1990)**
- ***Living Longer Stronger* (1995)**

- ***A Flat Stomach ASAP* (1998)**
- ***The New High-Intensity Training* (2004)**

Through my books and courses, I've built a following of people who trust my information.

I take that trust seriously. That's why all my guidelines and recommendations are based on scientific research and then tried and tested multiple times in real-world application on many different people. And it certainly helps if they continue to work year after year for many decades.

IronMan, *1972*

From age 15 to 40, I was very interested in bodybuilding and weight training. I exercised to have a bigger, better-shaped, and stronger body. During that time, from 1958 to 1983, I read a lot of what were called muscle magazines.

I read and reread *Strength & Health, IronMan, Muscular Development, Mr. America,* and *Muscle Builder* magazines. For me, the most interesting magazine—from the standpoint of providing honest, helpful routines and new techniques—was *IronMan.*

As I picked up my 1972 issue of *IronMan* from the mailbox, I thumbed through it quickly. *Hold it*—page 30 and page 31. Something caught my eye—and it was the word *negative.* The title of the article was "Accentuate the *Negative*" by Arthur Jones. I had read other articles by Jones, but this was the one I remember the best, even after more than 40 years.

Toward the end of the article, Jones challenged readers: "Start thinking in terms of *not* how much you can lift but, rather, how much you can lower." No lifter I knew of nor read about had ever thought about how much he could lower. It was always about how much you could lift.

That single article influenced me greatly, and it also influenced thousands and thousands of fitness-minded people.

I had met Jones 2 years earlier, in 1970, as he was in the process of starting Nautilus Sports/Medical Industries. Jones and Nautilus began to manufacture and market Nautilus strength-training machines, which were a radical departure from traditional barbells and dumbbells. I had visited Jones several times at his headquarters in Lake Helen, Florida. At that time, I was working on a PhD in exercise science at Florida State University in Tallahassee, which was about 225 miles north of Jones's headquarters.

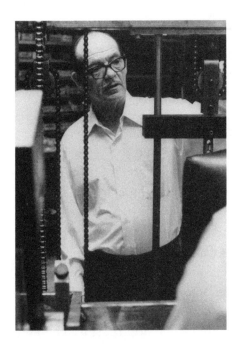

In the 1970s, Arthur Jones not only invented the Nautilus exercise machines—which required sprockets, chains, and weight stacks—but he also popularized a harder/briefer approach to training with barbells and dumbbells.

I got along well with Jones, which was something many people did not do, and I even told him that I'd like to work for Nautilus when I finished my research at Florida State.

A MUDDY EXPERIENCE

During one of my visits with Arthur, I showed him an article that I had written about exercising in a mud pit in Waco, Texas. A man I met in Waco had developed a series of mud exercises that he was using in a rectangular pit he had dug and coated with concrete near the Brazos River. The pit was filled with river-bottom clay, and you submerged yourself in the clay, which provided resistance against various body movements. I had trained in the mud pit several times, and I described what it was like in the magazine and also to Jones.

Jones quickly analyzed the movements and pointed out something to me that I had not considered. "The problem with mud resistance," Jones noted, "is that it provides no negative work. And without negative work, an exercise is of limited value."

Instantly, I realized Jones was right. Getting chin deep in mud requires a couple of tightly stretched horizontal ropes to hold you in place. Once in place, performing open-handed curls stresses the biceps, especially if you try to do them fast. For something similar, think of doing curls in water. Water supplies an easier version of the same physiology.

Once you contract your biceps and get to the top, there's no negative resistance on the lowering. If you really force your arm to extend, your triceps is the involved muscle. So mud (and water) exercise movements basically provide positive-only work.

Munich, Germany, 1972

A month later, I attended the scientific congress that preceded the 1972 Olympic Games in Munich, Germany. In one of the sessions, Paavo Komi, PhD, a Finnish physiologist, described how he had trained a small group of Scandinavian weight lifters by having them lower—not lift—heavier-than-normal barbells from overhead to the floor. He was confident that his negative training would provide these weight lifters with an edge in their approaching Olympic competition. Several days later, one of Komi's athletes won a gold medal, and two won bronzes.

I told Komi I was interested in his research and wanted to talk with him more. I also mentioned that I would soon be working with Arthur Jones of Nautilus Sports/Medical Industries. Komi shared with me that he'd experimented with various hydraulic machines to help with the lifting of very heavy barbells for his athletes, but the machines had been problematic.

When I flew back to Florida from Germany, I phoned Jones and told him about Komi and his research with negative work. "Bring those reports down to me," Jones replied.

FROM PROTOTYPE TO PRODUCTION

It took me about a month to break away and visit Jones, so I mailed Komi's research study to him for his inspection. When I returned to Jones's headquarters, I was surprised to learn that he and his prototyping team had built five functioning machines, which he called Omni. The Omni machines were big, bulky contraptions—and each one had a foot pedal that allowed the user to leg press the loaded weight stack to the top position. At the top position, you could grasp the movement arm with your hands and perform the negative position of the specific exercise with your arms and the upper-body muscles involved.

The advantage of such exercise was that it allowed you to load your upper-body muscles with a much heavier resistance than you could normally lift, without using your legs as a strong assistant. Believe me, this negative-training concept worked well enough that Nautilus manufactured and sold hundreds of the machines for a growing market.

Jones always pushed the idea of performing each repetition in a smooth, slow manner, with no quick or sudden movements. Properly performed negative exercise, Jones concluded, assured more complete exercise of the muscles because the resistance always moved at a steady pace and, as a result, provided more thorough stimulation of the muscle fibers. This was in contrast to the natural inclination to jerk and drop resistance, the manner in which a great deal of lifting was performed then and even now.

Negative-Training Drawbacks

First is the problem that you can't exercise your legs in this manner—and trying to use your arms to assist your legs doesn't work well. What you can do is get a couple of strong training partners to help you do the lifting of the movement arm on the various leg exercises, such as the leg curl and the leg press, as you use a heavier-than-normal amount of resistance. Your spotters must be careful at the top to transfer the load smoothly to your legs. Such lifting soon becomes tedious for even the most motivated assistants.

Second is the problem of your own strength. You will quickly become very strong from negative work. As a result, you may need another strong spotter to help you do the foot-pedal lifting. Again, that usually leads to an ongoing situation of trying to find a willing spotter.

Third is the problem of accurately judging the intensity of your negative repetitions. You can easily lapse into resting too long between repetitions.

A lag time of only 3 seconds allows your muscles a significant degree of recovery. Rather than becoming stronger, you are increasing resistance by lowering intensity.

Fourth, it can become dangerous if you rest too long between repetitions. A 3-second or longer rest or lag time between repetitions means that you are performing a series of single-attempt efforts. Such lifting can lead to poor form and possible injury.

THE MACHINE STALEMATE

As the years went by, Jones was in a quandary over designing machines with significantly more resistance on the negative stroke than on the positive stroke. He made many attempts—first, the Omni machines, which supplied a foot pedal to lift a heavier-than-normal resistance with the legs and then lower it with the arms; and last, with his servo-electrical machines that could be computer programmed to supply more resistance on the negative. Jones's endeavors provided benefits, but the machines were cumbersome and complex.

Jones sold Nautilus in 1986 and later retired from his follow-up company, MedX, in 1996. He died in 2007, having never solved how to construct an exercise machine with more negative than positive resistance.

You had to really understand what you were doing with negative training for it to be beneficial for more than 2 months. Fortunately, at the Nautilus headquarters, a few guys kept the fires burning, as you'll learn in the next chapter.

Mr. America Makes a Comeback

Learning from failure

I began work, officially, at Nautilus Sports/Medical Industries in July 1973. I had finished a PhD in exercise science at Florida State University in 1972 and stayed around for another year and a half doing a postdoctoral study in the food and nutrition department. I met Harold Schendel, PhD, of that department in 1969, and he impressed me with his knowledge and the work he had done in protein metabolism. Over several years, we explored the interplay between nutrition and building muscle.

What I learned with Schendel enters into the point of this chapter: the training of a bodybuilder named Casey Viator.

Casey Viator

Casey Viator worked for Nautilus and Arthur Jones for approximately 5 years—and those years were split into three periods.

1. **July 1970 through June 1971:** Jones trained Viator for the 1971 AAU Mr. America Contest, which he won in sensational style. Viator left after his win.

2. **March 1973 through March 1975:** Viator was injured in January 1973 and lost about 30 pounds. Jones rehired him, took him to Colorado State University, and put him through a grueling 28-day training period. This study became known as the Colorado Experiment. After 2 years, Viator left again.

3. **October 1977 through December 1978:** Viator returned to Nautilus a third time and then moved on.

I've written extensively in several of my books (including *The New High-Intensity Training*, 2004) about Viator winning the Mr. America contest. The rest of this chapter covers the third period in Viator's history at Nautilus.

The "Genetic Freak"

Arthur Jones often referred to Viator as a genetic freak in that he inherited exceptionally long muscle bellies and short tendon attachments throughout his body. These long muscles and short tendons provided him with the potential to build a huge amount of muscular size and strength in his forearms, upper arms, chest, lower back, thighs, and calves. Furthermore, he could do that quickly.

Jones enjoyed trying various techniques and routines on Viator because he could observe the results after only one or two workouts. For example, Viator—from one of Jones's workouts—could put half an inch on his contracted upper arm.

When Jones trained Viator, you could literally see him grow workout by workout. Unfortunately, the opposite was also true. When Viator trained himself, he got smaller and weaker. And few people would dare train Viator, because he was Mr. America—and supposedly, he knew all the ins and outs of training and bodybuilding.

So when Viator was hired for the third time, Jones turned him over to me for a project. Both Jones and I were interested in the concept of building muscle on a low-calorie diet. Viator had never been a big eater, so he agreed to drop his dietary calories to 1,800 a day. Usually he consumed about 3,600 calories daily.

On October 15, 1977, 26-year-old Viator stood 5 feet 8 inches tall and weighed 186 pounds. I was to train Viator 3 times a week on 12 Nautilus machines for 10 consecutive weeks. Viator performed a single set of 8 to 12 repetitions on each machine. Anytime he did 12 or more repetitions in good form, we increased the resistance at the next workout.

Concerning Viator's eating plan, he was instructed to consume 1,800 calories each day, divided into three 600-calorie meals.

Just for the record: Viator had previously weighed more than 200 pounds at several times during his employment at Nautilus. For example, he weighed 218 pounds when he won Mr. America in 1971, and he weighed 206 after he finished the Colorado Experiment in 1973. Thus, any muscle that he added during this 10-week program was probably muscle he was rebuilding. It's a physiological fact that it's easier to rebuild muscle than it is to build it.

Take a close look at the before-and-after photos of Viator. Over a 10-week period—October 15 through December 24, 1977—his strength on the 12 basic

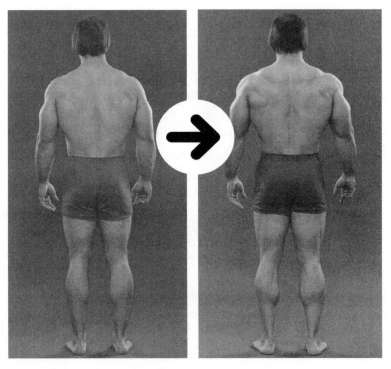

Over 10 weeks, while consuming only 1,800 calories per day,
Casey Viator packed on 23.43 pounds of muscle.

exercises increased by 28 percent. As a muscle gets stronger, its size and mass increase in almost direct proportion. Thus, his body weight went from 186 pounds to 206 pounds, a gain of 20 pounds, or 2 pounds per week.

Over that 10-week period, Viator lost 3.43 pounds of body fat. So his muscle gain was actually 23.43 pounds. You should be able to observe that Viator is definitely leaner in the after photo.

For Viator to build 23.43 pounds of muscle—on 1,800 calories a day, which was probably at or below his daily resting metabolic rate—his body had to resort to his fat stores as a source of calories to build muscle.

The Journey to the Mr. Universe Contest

By January 1, 1978, Casey Viator was rounding back into the shape and condition that he was in when he won Mr. America in 1971. He weighed a solid 206 pounds, but that was not enough. Jones's goal was to get Viator up to 220 before he entered the 1978 National Amateur Body-Builders' Association's Mr. Universe contest, held each year in August in London, England.

Jones, Viator, and I—plus Jim Flanagan—met in early January to map out our strategy for Viator. Flanagan owned a Nautilus Fitness Center in Orlando, which he managed at night, but he spent most weekdays at the Nautilus headquarters helping on the business side of the operation.

Jones knew that his motivation to train Viator consistently wouldn't last for more than a month, much less 8 months, so he wanted Flanagan and me to supervise Viator's weekly training. We all knew that to be successful, we were going to have to hit Viator with some heavy negative exercise at least once a week for most of the next 8 months. Sure, we could still use the basic routines that I'd applied in my 10-week plan. But adding 15 pounds of muscle to Viator's body wasn't going to come easy. We had to combine the basic routines with our best negative techniques.

Flanagan and I worked overtime coming up with a variety of routines, most of which involved negatives on the following Nautilus machines: hip and back, leg press, pullover, decline press, overhead press, biceps, triceps, and the negative-only chin and dip on the multiexercise machine.

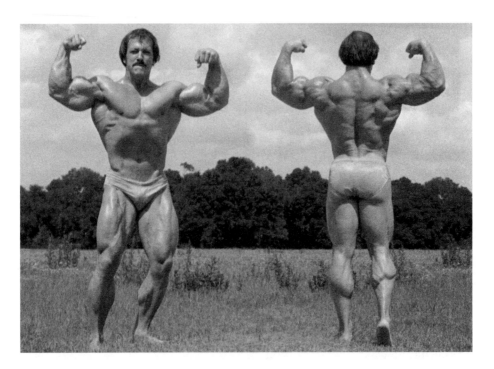

Six months of hard training, and approximately 50 percent of it performed in a negative-
accentuated manner, increased Viator's body weight from 206 to 224 pounds.
That was a gain of 18 pounds of solid muscle. In my opinion, Viator was in his best-ever shape.

Viator made nice progress. At the end of May, we reduced his intense workouts per week from three to two. Doing that seemed to invigorate Viator, as
well as both Flanagan and me.

On July 18, 1978, I took these front-and-back photos of Viator posing in a
field near the Nautilus headquarters. He weighed 224 pounds, which exceeded
our goal of 220 pounds by 4 pounds. Now we were building areas of his body
that lay dormant before. That was also a gain of 18 pounds since our first
workout in mid-January.

Viator looked unbeatable in the condition he was in on that July morning.
And we still had a month of training left.

For whatever reason, during August, we all seemed to take at least some of
the training for granted. Maybe we should have reduced his frequency again.

When Viator, Flanagan, and I—plus our wives—arrived in London, Viator had
lost some of his size—and his swagger. It was obvious to me from his showing in

the morning's prejudging that Viator weighed less than 220 pounds, probably closer to 215 pounds. He was overanxious and probably dehydrated. As a result, he placed second to Dave Johns in the 1978 Mr. Universe contest.

Looking back on the situation, Viator peaked a month too soon.

WHAT WE LEARNED

The Casey Viator project taught me several lessons that I considered as I designed the Body Fat Breakthrough program:

→ Plan well from the beginning.

→ Stick to basic routines most of the time.

→ Rebuild muscle and lose fat, or build muscle and lose fat. You can do the condition that applies to you on a reduced-calorie diet, because nutrition is secondary to growth stimulation.

→ Introduce negative training gradually, even with gifted athletes.

→ Don't overdo negative training.

→ Decrease your training frequency as your strength and conditioning improve.

→ Learn from your success. Learn even more from your failure.

CHAPTER 9

Nautilus and the New Machine

Every decade, new techniques and technologies emerge that have been inspired by past success

IF you can do something you like for a living, going to work each day is as good as it gets.

That's exactly how I felt each day I went to work for Arthur Jones and Nautilus Sports/Medical Industries. And it lasted 20 years.

My rebuilding and building experiences with Casey Viator opened the door to apply this knowledge to regular people who aren't bodybuilders. I liked to write, and Arthur Jones did not. It wasn't that Jones couldn't write. In fact, he was the best composer of words that I've ever met. His problem was that writing was too easy for him.

If you could make Jones sit down in front of a typewriter and get one sentence out of him, it just flowed, sentence after sentence, page after page. Jones could hardly stop it.

The problem was that you could not get him to sit down often enough at a typewriter.

Words didn't flow out of my typewriter like they did out of Jones's, but my motivation, frequency, and consistency made up for it. Plus, Jones encouraged my research and writing.

As the popularity of fitness, strength training, and Nautilus equipment increased throughout the United States, so did my opportunities for articles and books on these subjects.

At first I became involved in producing a series of small paperbound books, which included *Strength-Training Principles* (published 1977), *How to Lose Body Fat* (1977), *How Your Muscles Work: Featuring Nautilus Equipment* (1978), *Nutrition for Athletes* (1978), and *Conditioning for Football* (1979). We sold those little books by the hundreds, mostly to Nautilus Fitness Centers, where they were used as promotional items for members and prospective members.

Then I did four books that were sold in traditional bookstores and sporting goods stores throughout the United States. I had a couple of bestsellers in this group; namely, *The Nautilus Book* (1980) and *The Nautilus Bodybuilding Book* (1982). Both were filled with elegant photos of each Nautilus machine and techniques for using it properly. I was pleased when, in July 1984, *The Nautilus Bodybuilding Book* was listed in the number one position of the American Booksellers Association, paperback division. Ranked under my book were *The New Aerobics* by Kenneth Cooper and *The Inner Game of Tennis* by Timothy Gallwey.

The popularity of bodybuilding was soaring. Luckily for me, while in London at the 1978 Mr. Universe contest, I had met Chris Lund. Lund was considered by many to be the best bodybuilding photographer in the world. His specialty was black-and-white, as he did all his own darkroom work.

Lund and I teamed up to do a series of large-format books for Perigee/Putnam. Again, there were a number of bestsellers, such as *High-Intensity Bodybuilding* (1984), *Super High-Intensity Bodybuilding* (1986), and *Massive Muscles in 10 Weeks* (1987).

Besides my book writing, there was a lot going on at Nautilus. Jones was constantly redesigning his Nautilus machines and making them more efficient. Besides the Omni machines, he had several machines he called Duo-Poly, and then he introduced the Duo-Squat machine. Then there was Infimetric exercising, Leverage Plate-Loading, and Computerized Lumbar-Testing equipment.

Jim Flanagan was busy organizing Nautilus seminars. Jones had constructed a big complex behind the front offices that now housed a couple of showrooms, TV studios, and a multifunctional auditorium that could seat 300 people. Jones's instruction to Flanagan was, "Every other month, fill those seats with people—people who want to purchase Nautilus equipment and people who want to learn how to use the equipment properly." Flanagan welcomed that challenge for years and was successful in fulfilling it.

Flanagan and I both traveled 20 weekends per year, as Nautilus was a sponsor for the Medalist High School Coaching Clinics. At those clinics we shared the Nautilus strength-training philosophy with high school coaches throughout the United States, and we got to rub shoulders with the NCAA Championship coaches from the previous year's football and basketball seasons.

The Importance of Trust

In 1984, Nautilus was booming. Close by, in Gainesville, Florida, where the University of Florida is located, Joe Cirulli was quietly operating one of the best-run fitness centers in the world. He and a dozen members of his staff always attended our fitness seminars. In his club, Cirulli had 18,000 members, six lines of Nautilus machines, and several qualified instructors on each line. Thousands and thousands of people were exercising at Cirulli's club daily. Most important, each person was strength training effectively and efficiently.

Talking with Cirulli and seeing his club in operation prompted me to come up with a plan whereby together we could place overfat people on a strength-training program, as well as on a lower-calorie diet, and supervise them through a several-month program. I called the program the Nautilus Diet. That was the birth of an alliance and friendship between Cirulli and me that is still going strong.

In 1987, with the publication of *The Nautilus Diet: 10 Weeks to a Brand-New Body,* I presented evidence that with proper strength training, it was possible to lose fat and build muscle simultaneously. That was the first time that concept had been demonstrated with a large group.

The popularity of building muscle to lose fat was high enough that the demand for similar how-to manuals was almost open-ended. From 1988 to 2004, I published 18 more books, including *The Six-Week Fat-to-Muscle Makeover* (1988), *Big Arms in Six Weeks* (1988), *BIG* (1990), *Hot Hips and Fabulous Thighs* (1991), *Body Defining* (1996), and *The New High-Intensity Training* (2004).

I explained negative-accentuated training in my listed books, but it was applied sparingly or not at all.

In most of my books, I supervised the dieting and exercising of participants from Gainesville. In fact, I have records, including before-and-after photos, of 519 women and 318 men, or a total of 837 members of Gainesville Health & Fitness (GHF) in various programs.

Negative-Accentuated Training: Building Muscle to Lose Fat

This vault of materials from Gainesville allowed me to analyze and compare more than 25 years of studies directly related to building muscle to lose fat. And perhaps most important, the eating plan in all my studies and books has remained basically the same: 50 percent carbohydrates, 25 percent fats, and 25 percent proteins. Only the strength-training routine has varied. For example, I may have applied Nautilus equipment, MedX, free-weight exercises, freehand movements, or even Bowflex machines.

Bottom line: I had never before been involved in a research project that reinforced the building-muscle-to-lose-fat concept—with such dramatic before-and-after data and photos—the way my 2012 negative-accentuated studies in Gainesville did.

I was director of research for Nautilus Sports/Medical Industries for 20 years and was involved with the Colorado Experiment, the West Point Study, Omni machines, Duo-Poly training, Infimetric exercising, Nautilus computerized machines, Duo-Squat machines, Leverage Plate-Loading systems, Computerized Lumbar-Testing equipment, and many other techniques, systems, trials, and tests.

Negative-accentuated exercise and my GHF training routines are more relevant today than any of the above-listed Nautilus developments. And negative-accentuated training has more fat-loss and muscle-building potential than any of the programs and courses published in my previous books.

Let the negative-accentuated reform begin.

Weight Stacks That Tilt

Enter a new machine from Stockholm.

A standard exercise machine like Nautilus equipment has a weight stack that moves in a vertical manner. It moves straight up during the positive phase and straight down during the negative.

If there's little or no friction on the guide rods and redirectional pulleys with 140 pounds on the weight stack, then the user has 140 pounds on the lifting and 140 pounds on the lowering.

But think about this: What if you could tilt the weight stack from the bottom to 45 degrees? Then, with a 45-degree tilt to the stack, 140 pounds moving diagonally would weigh approximately 100 pounds.

Now, as you finish lifting the resistance, what if you could instantly tilt the weight stack back to the vertical position? Then you'd be able to perform the negative with the original 140 pounds, or 40 percent more than you did on the diagonal, or pushing, phase of the lift.

This was the way Mats Thulin of Stockholm, Sweden, described his chest-press machine to me in a phone call in early October 2008. I had met Mats in 1980 at one of the Nautilus training seminars in Florida. He later became a distributor of Nautilus equipment in Scandinavia.

"Ellington," Thulin said, "I've developed a new way to accentuate the negative without the use of the legs or the involvement of an assistant. Please come to Sweden and have a look for yourself."

On November 13, 2008, I flew to Stockholm to meet with Thulin and try this new negative-accentuated equipment, which he had named X-Force. I wasn't disappointed.

In Stockholm, when I critically examined what Thulin had done and applied it under workout conditions, a clear message popped into my head. *Why didn't Arthur Jones or one of his engineers, or even I—think of this approach decades ago?*

The approach that Thulin applied so effectively involves a tilting weight stack powered by an electric servomotor. As the user begins the positive stroke, the weight stack is at a 45-degree angle. This angle reduces the selected resistance by approximately 29 percent. At the top of the positive stroke, the tilted weight stack returns to vertical. The user then lowers 100 percent of the selected resistance.

Instead of continuing to search for ways to add resistance on the negative, which was the strategy employed by Jones and others, Thulin figured out a way to subtract weight from the positive.

This was a brilliant step forward in the advancement of strength-training machines.

Reaching Failure Faster

While I exercised in Stockholm, two machines, the X-Force Leg Curl and the X-Force Biceps Curl, caught my attention. These machines, minus the tilting weight stacks, were almost identical to ones I had in my private gym in Florida. Perhaps I could make some valid comparisons between X-Force and my normal weight-stack machines?

On the X-Force Leg Curl and the X-Force Biceps Curl, I calculated and selected the same amount of resistance for the positive phases as I had used the week before in Florida. Each repetition, however, would supply 40 percent more resistance on the negative phase. My goal was to perform as many repetitions as possible, using a 2-second-positive and 4-second-negative count.

Interestingly, on both X-Force exercises, I barely completed 7 repetitions and reached momentary muscular failure at approximately 42 seconds. The week before, using my conventional leg curl and biceps curl machines, I had reached failure on each at 10 repetitions and 60 seconds.

This demonstrated to me that with these X-Force machines, I could achieve the same level of fatigue in 42 seconds, as opposed to 60 seconds. Thus, the X-Force Leg Curl and Biceps Curl machines, for me, were 50 percent more demanding per repetition and required 30 percent less time to

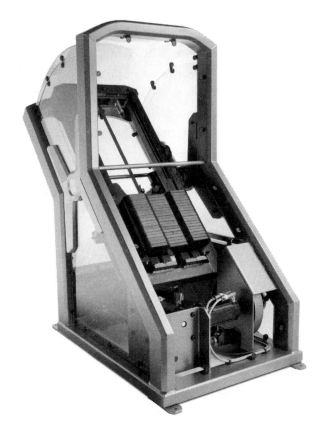

A cutaway of the back of an X-Force weight stack. Notice that the mechanism is tilted to 45 degrees. When the weight stack is angled, the resistance—as it is lifted—weighs significantly less. When the mechanism is tilted back to vertical, the resistance when lowering weighs 40 percent more than when it is angled. A servo-electrical motor at the bottom, with a sensor, moves the weight stack efficiently either way in half a second.

failure (42 seconds versus 60 seconds). More about the repetition-by-repetition demand of negative-accentuated training will be discussed in Chapter 14.

X-Force's concept has my vote for efficiency in action.

Stimulated to Grow

When I returned to my home in Florida, I was determined to figure out how to apply what I learned in Sweden to my standard equipment. It took me a while, but over the next 2 years, I tried, tested, retried, and unraveled, finally, the most important factor behind what Thulin had done with his X-Force machines.

Performing a heavy negative repetition on a traditional resistance-exercise machine involves a lag time, whereby a spotter has to help the user with the positive phase. During the lag time, the involved muscles, even though they are doing some of the lifting, are still resting to some unknown degree. X-Force, with its tilting weight stack, had effectively removed the lag time between repetitions. Why? Because the user had to do both the negative and the positive work—continuously and unassisted.

After a couple of X-Force repetitions, the resistance on the negative was near maximum, and the resistance on the positive was also near maximum. So it became a struggle, a real struggle but not an impossibility, to perform the last positive and then the last negative. If you performed your set in that manner, your involved muscles felt as though they were actually being stimulated to grow toward the end of the set.

That feeling, in my opinion, was the key. But again, why? Because that "stimulated to grow" feeling was an indication that those key hormones—MGF, IL-6, IGF-1, GH, and IL-15—described in Chapter 4 had been activated. Getting those hormones into the bloodstream was essential for the fat-loss and muscle-gain breakthrough that I was searching for.

So my task was simply: How do I simulate that feeling with a Nautilus machine or any standard exercise machine that has a vertical weight stack?

The solution may not surprise you—since I've already leaked, several times, the answer: the 30-30-30 technique. A discussion of it follows in the next chapter.

CHAPTER 10

30–30–30

The new cadence for the negative, positive, negative phases yields greater gains

TO achieve positive and near-maximum negative . . . in the same set of an exercise. That was my goal.

Actually, Jim Flanagan started me thinking about this challenge. Flanagan, the former general manager at the Nautilus headquarters, also joined me in the training of Casey Viator back in 1978. Today, he lives about 20 miles from me. We both have private gyms in our homes, and we have clients who visit us weekly for personal training.

In early 2011, Flanagan decided to try a few "hypers" with some of his trainees. Hypers, a term coined by Arthur Jones, involve loading a strength-training machine with 40 percent more resistance than a trainee would normally do for 10 repetitions, which will be just right for 6 or 7 good negative repetitions. A spotter or helper assists the lifter just enough to make the positive feel near maximum for the 6 or 7 repetitions but does not assist during the negative part of the exercise.

With a little practice from both the spotter and the trainee, the situation becomes a set performed with near-maximum positive resistance and near-maximum negative resistance. If you know anything about strength training, you should be able to see that hyper repetitions, if you worked them just right using five or six consecutive machines, would be a heck of a workout.

Flanagan was telling me about doing hypers with some of his strongest men, most of whom are ex-football players. And he had gotten some of them to help him work out in the same style.

Believe me, I've seen Jim Flanagan train, and he's well into his sixties. Flanagan handles a lot of resistance. When he trains, which is not very often (once every 10 days), he trains heavy, very heavy.

After Flanagan trained himself with hypers, he called to tell me about how sore he was—sore to the point that he had trouble sitting on the toilet and even more difficulty getting back up.

So I decided to try hypers with some of my trainees and, in turn, gave it a try myself. And Flanagan was right. Sitting was a problem for us, too, and it lasted for several days!

The Problem with Hypers

Doing hypers is filled with other problems. First, the spotting has to be done precisely and carefully, which is difficult. Even those experienced at spotting can easily help on the positive too much or too little. Either way detracts from the overall goal of what you're trying to do.

Second, when you're spotting, exactly how do you know if you are assisting just the right amount? You don't, unless you've had a whole lot of experience. Third, if you have had plenty of experience with hypers, you are probably not fond of them, because you must to do a lot of lifting, twisting, and straining—with one arm or one leg.

Hypers are interesting from the standpoint that they could go into the toolbox of an advanced trainer or trainee, where they could be applied occasionally. But they are not practical for more casual exercisers.

Nevertheless, Jim Flanagan and his hypers got me to thinking that there had to be something similar but safer. There was . . . and it was connected to a style of training that I've applied many times, even on a weekly basis in my private gym.

Extremely S-L-O-W Repetitions

In the spring of 1999, I posted an article on my Web site, DrDarden.com, under the title "Extremely S-L-O-W Repetitions." In this article, I discussed how, some 20 years earlier at Nautilus, we tried working up to 60 seconds on the positive and 60 seconds on the negative in two exercises: the chinup and the dip. Later I used these exercises in several arm routines, which I included in two of my bodybuilding books.

In fact, if you've ever tried any of my advanced arm routines that involved this extremely slow style, you were probably awed at the effects of a very slow chinup and a slow dip. They definitely work.

Since 2002, I've had a private gym in my home. The gym is small and contains five Nautilus Nitro machines, a Bowflex machine, a barbell, two dumbbells, and an early Nautilus Multi-Exercise machine that I use primarily for the chinup, dip, and calf raise.

At first I added variety to my basic machines and exercises by introducing extremely slow chinups and dips to my stronger trainees. The way to do a slow chin, for example, is to start on the negative. Grasp the overhead bar with an underhand grip and your hands shoulder-width apart. Climb the stairs of the multi-exercise machine. Get your chin over the bar with your elbows beside your torso. Ease your feet from the step, steady your body, and slowly begin lowering your chin, head, shoulders, and legs all the way down until your arms are fully extended.

A 30-second lowering time is required before a trainee attempts a regular positive chin, from the bottom to the top, in 2 seconds.

The goal is to eventually get strong enough to perform a 30-second positive, followed by a 30-second negative. That's 1 repetition in 60 seconds.

Then, if you really want a challenge, try working up to a 60-second positive immediately followed by a 60-second negative. When you can do that, you probably won't need my book or my help.

After a year or so, I added the extremely slow style to the leg press, chest press, and a few other machine exercises. Quickly, I could see that the repetitions work best with long-range-of-movement exercises. They don't apply well to short-range exercises, such as the calf raise and wrist curl.

They also apply best to machines, as opposed to barbell and dumbbell (or free-weight) exercises. With most barbell and dumbbell exercises, there are natural sticking points when you're moving straight up against gravity that are not well suited for slow training. A properly designed exercise machine can compensate for the sticking point by smoothing out the resistance curve.

Negative, Positive, Negative

It was early one morning in January 2011. I was in my private gym and thinking about X-Force, hyper training, and extremely slow repetitions. If the negative phase of an exercise is more important than the positive, why don't I focus not on doing more weight but on doing more negative time than positive time?

I had already done this occasionally on the chin-up, dip, and leg press. To explore what I was getting at, the order had to be negative, positive, negative, which would be $1\frac{1}{2}$ repetitions.

That morning I tried various versions: 15 seconds for each phase, then 20 seconds, 30 seconds, and 40 seconds.

Then I tried two and three cycles of $1\frac{1}{2}$ repetitions in the same set, with an exact number of seconds per phase, and I compared the kinesthetic feel.

Wow, I thought to myself. *I'm on to a style that may be of real value.*

I believe in taking my time in exploring new techniques. I began trying various versions of the negative-positive-negative style with my most experienced trainees. After several months of applying, recording, and comparing, I then brought in some beginning trainees. And I did the same comparisons with them.

By the fall of 2011, I was ready to share what I was doing with Jim Flanagan. I knew Flanagan would give it a good trial with some of his big, strong ex-football players . . . which he did.

Flanagan and I kicked around a couple of variations, and he concurred with me and my procedures.

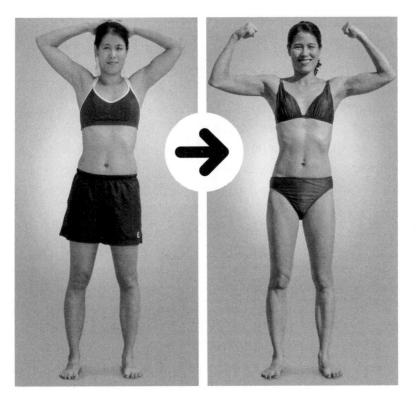

Dr, Roxanne Achong-Coan, 41, was one of my Orlando trainees who helped test my negative-accentuated ideas. After 8 weeks on my program, she lost 17.4 pounds of fat and built 6.4 pounds of muscle.

Here's what I concluded:

→ The ideal repetition format is a 30-second negative, followed by a 30-second positive, immediately followed by a final 30-second negative. And you must be able to do that with 80 percent of the resistance that you can handle for a regular set of 8 to 12 repetitions to failure.

→ Remember, the ideal repetition format involves approximately twice as much negative work as positive work. That's twice as much time: 60 seconds on the negative versus 30 seconds on the positive. Time, not resistance, is the key to procedure.

→ Negative training makes you very strong. The resistance you can use on a machine increases rapidly. Time, rather than resistance, makes it simpler for the trainee and the spotter. Plus, after the trainee gets the hang of the procedure, he may be able to do the workout himself, without a spotter, by doing the opening positive quickly.

Points to Consider

When doing negative, positive, negative training, keep these important points in mind:

→ It's best to have a spotter help you initially. In a machine exercise, the spotter assists in getting the movement arm to the top position. Then, while looking at a watch or a big clock with a second hand, he gives you a running count on your first negative half repetition of 5 seconds, 10 seconds, 15 seconds (halfway down), 20 seconds, 25 seconds, and 30 seconds (turn around the movement and start a positive) . . . 5 seconds, 10 seconds, 15 seconds (halfway up), 20 seconds, 25 seconds, and 30 seconds (turn around the movement and begin a finish negative) . . . 5 seconds, 10 seconds, 15 seconds (halfway down), 20 seconds, 25 seconds, and 30 seconds . . . smoothly stop.

→ Your spotter also has to be attentive to your slow movements. If you get stuck (it will probably occur initially during the positive), your helper needs to assist you just enough to get you through a certain range of motion, and then back off. Be sure to accurately record your

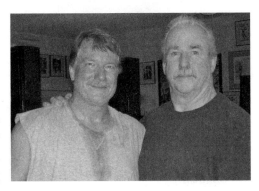

Floyd Scholz (*left*) was the strongest trainee involved with 30–30–30 testing. Scholz was the 1979 NCAA Decathlon Champion, and today, at 55 years of age, he has a rare combination of extraordinary strength and endurance. This photo was taken within 2 minutes after he finished one of his 30-30-30 workouts, which was supervised by Jim Flanagan (*right*).

stoppage. For example: If you did 30 seconds on the negative, 22 seconds on the positive, and 30 seconds on the negative, your notation on your workout sheet would be 30-22-30. When you can finally achieve 30-30-30, increase the resistance by 5 to 10 percent at your next workout.

→ Proper breathing is essential for success with slow repetitions. The key to proper breathing is to take short, shallow breaths. You should emphasize exhalation more than inhalation, especially during the finish negative. It's especially important that you don't hold your breath.

→ The 30-30-30 technique is adaptable to many body weight movements. They will be illustrated and described in Chapter 16, along with free-weight and machine exercises.

BEFORE-AND-AFTER PROOF

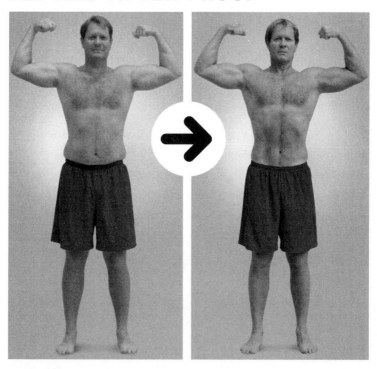

Dr. Max Medary, 47, has trained with me for 5 years. During this time, I've put him through many negative-accentuated sessions. Over a 1-year period, during 2010 and 2011, Medary lost 31.7 pounds of fat and built 11.7 pounds of muscle.

Six of my personal coaching trainees progressed through some of my negative-positive-negative, 30-30-30 routines at my private gym in Orlando during 2011. Dr. Max Medary's before-and-after photos are shown opposite, and Dr. Roxanne Achong-Coan's were featured earlier in this chapter. My wife Jeanenne's before-and-after comparisons are displayed in Chapter 13. I felt well prepared in 2012 to experiment with my new version of negative-accentuated training with some of Joe Cirulli's interested Gainesville Health & Fitness members.

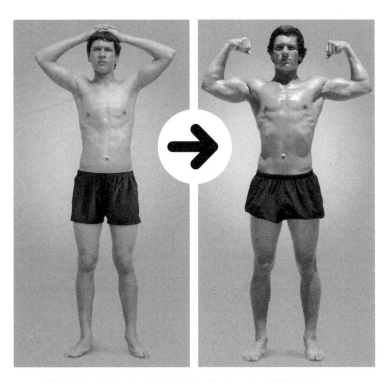

Chris Medary, 14, trained with his father Max throughout 2011. Chris grew 2 inches in height and added 30.5 pounds of solid muscle. Some of Chris's muscular gains were due to his normal maturation process.

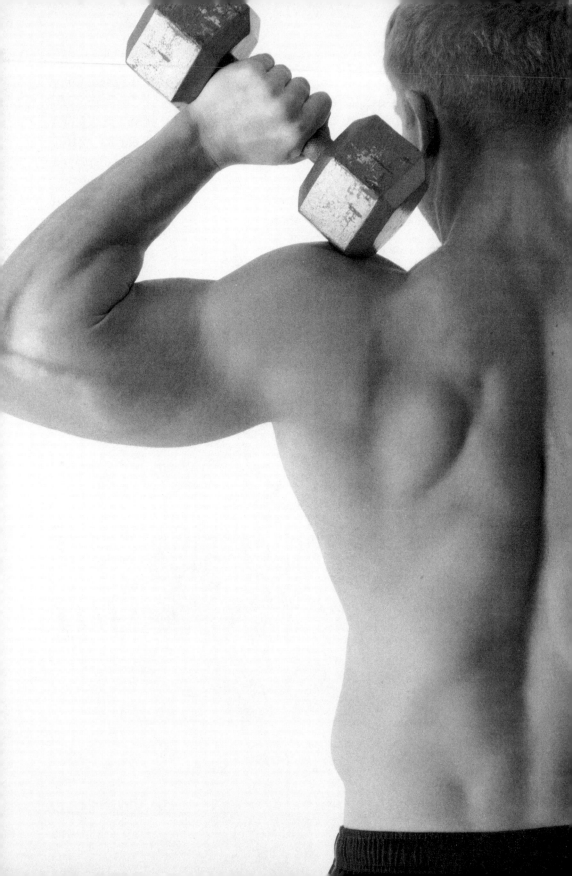

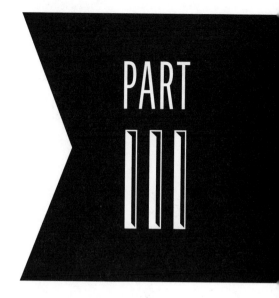

The Science of Negative-Accentuated Training

STORM ROBERTS
BEFORE & AFTER

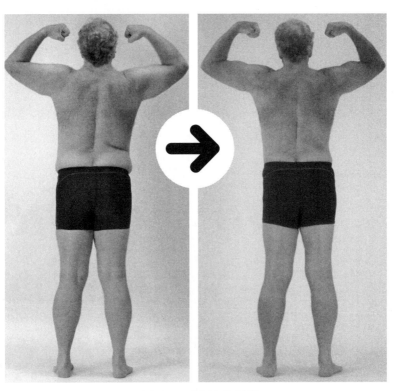

AGE 61, HEIGHT 6'0"

BEFORE BODY WEIGHT

256.86
POUNDS

AFTER BODY WEIGHT

202
POUNDS

AFTER 15 WEEKS

65.67
POUNDS OF FAT LOSS

9.5
INCHES OFF WAIST

10.81
POUNDS OF MUSCLE GAIN

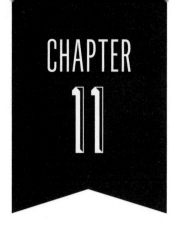

Reasons to Accentuate the Negative

A physics lesson that leads to a stronger, more muscular body—guaranteed

"The simplest definition of science is the search for rules."

—CARL SAGAN

CARL Sagan thought people who found everyday experiences a muddled jumble of events with no predictability and no regularity were in grave danger. The vast, exciting universe that Sagan wrote about belonged to people whose lives were governed by principles, rules, and guidelines.

While I don't claim to have it all figured out about fat loss, I have much experience in instructing and directing groups of overfat men and women to achieve leaner, stronger bodies. In the process of doing that for more than 4 decades, I've assembled meaningful rules related to exercising, eating, losing fat, and building muscular size and strength, as well as troubleshooting and maintenance.

In the next chapters, you'll learn some definitions and reasons to accentuate the negative. Plus, you'll understand the science of making deeper inroads with negative training.

You'll soon be prepared to apply the recommended negative-accentuated principles and exercises and see the results for yourself.

I've used the words *positive* and *negative* many times already. But what does each term really mean, and how does each tie in to muscular biomechanics?

A Few Definitions

Performing a strength-training exercise using a machine or a barbell requires the raising and lowering of resistance against the linear force of gravity. When you raise the selected resistance on the weight stack, you're moving vertically against gravity and performing positive work, or, in the language of physiologists, concentric muscle action is occurring. Lowering the weight involves controlling gravitational pull and is called negative work, or eccentric muscle action. During positive work, your muscle fibers are shortening. During negative work, the same fibers are lengthening. In the simplest terms, observing the weight stack move during an exercise reveals: Up is positive, down is negative.

(Note: In physics, *positive* and *negative* are terms that refer to the resistance, or external load. While these terms are not always technically correct in their applications in this book, their interchangeable use—**positive = concentric** and **negative = eccentric**—is overwhelmingly accepted by trainees, coaches, and athletes.)

When I started training with weights as a teenager in 1959, no one paid any attention to the negative phase of an exercise. Using mostly barbells and dumbbells, we performed the positive part of each repetition in a reasonable manner. The negative phase, however, was done haphazardly. Sometimes the weight was simply dropped.

Generally, most individuals who strength trained back then didn't give the negative any thought at all. They just focused on the lifting.

I trained that way until 1972. That was when I read the article by Arthur Jones in *IronMan* magazine that I discussed in Chapter 7. Today, I know that it was a waste to not take the negative part of a repetition seriously. The physics of the situation will help you understand why.

The Physics of Positive and Negative Work

Research with positive and negative work reveals that strength training obeys the basic physical laws described centuries ago by Isaac Newton. Newton's law of inertia states that an object at rest tends to stay at rest unless acted upon by an outside force. This applies directly to the lifting of a weight at the start of a concentric (positive) muscle action.

For example, in the standing barbell curl, the weight begins at rest with the biceps muscle ready to act. If the muscular force exceeds the inertia of the barbell, movement occurs and the barbell is lifted. Concentric muscle action, therefore, is used to initiate, maintain, or increase motion of an object.

An eccentric muscle action has a different effect. In Newton's law of acceleration, an object that is already in motion tends to stay in motion unless acted on by an outside force. In strength training, an object that has been raised by concentric muscle action is now pulled back by the force of gravity. Only with muscular force exerted against the descending weight can it be prevented from accelerating downward.

Concentric and eccentric muscle actions have evolved to accommodate the laws of motion. Muscle force during shortening is less than force during lengthening because it is harder to create a new bond than to break an existing bond.

The process of shortening is complex, energy dependent, and based on creating new chemical bonds within the muscle. But once formed, these bonds are extremely stable and thus make the lengthening process so appropriate for overloading. That's why a person can become stronger quickly with progressively heavier and heavier negative resistance.

In other words, the stability of the existing chemical bonds involved in lowering a heavy resistance reacts appropriately and adapts well to the right negative-accentuated training, combined with more than adequate rest and sleep.

10 Reasons to Accentuate the Negative

Here are the beneficial actions of negative or eccentric exercise, according to the scientific literature:

→ Involves a heavier-than-normal overload—which means more force output and more muscle fibers recruited

→ Recruits more fast-twitch fibers—which contribute predominantly to muscular size

→ Ensures a higher level of stress per motor unit—which supplies greater stimulation of the involved muscle fibers

→ Requires greater neural adaptation—which reinforces cross-education of strength gains from one limb or side to the other

→ Causes more microscopic fiber tears—which ignite the muscle-building process

→ Works the entire joint structure—which results in more strength, stability, range of motion, and healing properties

→ Applies well to postsurgical therapy—which is advantageous in rehabilitation

→ Maintains strength gains longer—which counters the detraining process

→ Transfers strength gains to positive work—which is valuable in lifting performance

→ Allows greater work in less time—which means more efficient training sessions and faster results

And there's a huge benefit, which may be the most important of all. Negative training makes a deeper inroad, repetition by repetition, throughout the entire set—which stimulates the production of growth hormone (GH), insulin-like growth factor 1 (IGF-1), mechano-growth factor (MGF), interleukin 6 (IL-6), and interleukin 15 (IL-15). All these chemicals pulsating into the bloodstream not only lead to muscle hypertrophy but also oxidize fat-cell content at a faster-than-normal rate.

Rapid release of fat is probably assisted by a related hormone's anabolic influence on both muscle and fat. That hormone is insulin. Apparently, intense negative-accentuated training decreases the effect of insulin on fat and increases the effect of insulin on muscle.

In other words, with negative-accentuated training, the deeper inroad diminishes insulin sensitivity among fat cells, and they begin to shrink. As insulin sensitivity in the muscle elevates, glucose and nutrients are directed preferentially into muscle cells, and they expand.

Expanded muscle cells and shrunken fat cells equals more muscle and less fat. More muscle and less fat equals a stronger, leaner, better-shaped body.

Negative-accentuated training, by stimulating and directing the body's natural hormones, provides a new way to build muscle and lose fat quickly.

Styles of Negative Training

There are a number of ways to accentuate the negative during an exercise.

1. On a leg curl machine, lift the resistance with both legs, and then lower with only one leg supporting the resistance. Lift again with both legs and lower with the other. Then alternate the lowering legs for 5 or 6 repetitions of each leg. The idea here is to use 70 percent of the resistance that you would normally apply for the standard leg curl. Lowering 70 percent of your regular weight with one leg is equivalent to lowering 140 percent with both legs.

The problem with this style is that one leg is always resting, which inhibits growth stimulation.

2. Use an experienced spotter to add more resistance during the lower-ing or negative stage of the lift. For example, the trainee on the leg curl machine could lift the resistance with both legs and the spotter could add more force during the lowering by pushing down on the roller pad. The key to best results is a slow, deliberate lowering of the

heavier-than-normal movement arm, with no sudden drops. Try this style for 8 to 10 repetitions.

The problem with this style is getting an experienced spotter to manage the lowering repetitions. Even with an experienced spotter, it is difficult to record accurately what happens during a set.

3. Again with an experienced spotter, you could load the machine with 30 to 40 percent more resistance than normal and do the hyper style, which was described on page 66. In the hyper style, the spotter helps with the positive, but just enough to keep the resistance arm moving. Then the trainee guides the heavier negative slowly to the bottom and repeats for 6 or 7 more repetitions.

The problem, once again, is finding an experienced spotter. Also, hypers are not practical over a lengthy period of time.

4. Computer-programmed machines, such as Milon of Germany and Exerbotics of the United States, provide an electrical form of resistance that is programmed heavier on the negative phase. Other machines, such as MaxOut of the United States and X-Force of Sweden, use electrical motors to either add resistance on the negative or tilt the weight stack on the positive. Both types of machines supply 40 percent more resistance on the negative phase of each repetition.

The problem with the machines of Milon, Exerbotics, and MaxOut is that they are not smooth. They tend to be jerky to the point that their kinesthetic feel is simply *not right.*

X-Force is the only negative-accentuated equipment that is on target. But it has only recently become available in Europe and is not being actively marketed in the United States. The potential for X-Force, however, is great. For detailed information about this equipment, see the Appendix.

5. On almost any exercise performed with your body weight, a barbell, dumbbells, or a machine, you can make the negative phase harder by moving slower. The most recommended guideline to apply here is 2-4: That's 2 seconds on the positive, followed by 4 seconds on the lowering.

The problem with the 2-4 method is that it's too easy to cheat on the counting, so it turns into the standard way of training: up and down to the same beat.

What Actually Works: 30-30-30

The five methods that I describe above all have problems and, while many of the problems have solutions, solving them may not be worth the time, effort, and money involved.

Since X-Force is not widely available, I believe that the best method is the style that I developed in 2011 and further refined in 2012 . . . called 30-30-30. To perform properly, take 80 percent of the weight you'd normally handle for 8 to 12 repetitions and do a 30-second negative, followed by a 30-second positive, followed by a final 30-second negative. That's $1\frac{1}{2}$ repetitions, or 60 seconds of negative work and 30 seconds of positive work. Actually, the half repetitions may vary between 20 and 30 seconds on each segment.

The problem with 30-30-30 is that, for at least several weeks, it's best to have a spotter assist you on the first half repetitions. Also, the spotter needs a watch with a second hand, so he/she can pace you with the lowering and lifting half repetitions. With a good spotter or training partner, this problem can be overcome.

The 30-30-30 style is the best way to accentuate the negative. It's safe, precise, and productive. Yes, you can become very strong with this method. But you won't need extremely heavy weights, as you do with hypers.

Furthermore, the slow style may actually temporarily shut down some of the blood flow to and from the working muscles. If this is the case, there's Japanese research that shows that occluded muscles, once released, overcompensate to a greater degree than muscles that are not occluded. Thus, the 30-30-30 type of occlusion may be another way that the growth process is stimulated.

The next chapter supplements the negative-accentuated growth process by connecting it with the concept of *inroad*. This is a key idea to understand.

KATHERINE HERRING
BEFORE & AFTER

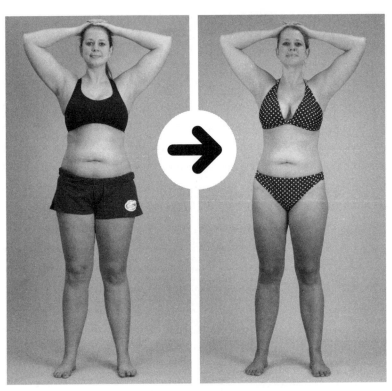

AGE 29, HEIGHT 5'8.5"

BEFORE BODY WEIGHT

197
POUNDS

AFTER BODY WEIGHT

167
POUNDS

AFTER 12 WEEKS

37.32
POUNDS OF FAT LOSS

5.25
INCHES OFF WAIST

7.32
POUNDS OF MUSCLE GAIN

CHAPTER 12

Recognizing the Power of "Inroad"

Why anything less than high-intensity effort is a waste of your time

IT'S time to really understand *inroad* and its importance in building muscle.

An inroad, by definition, is the depletion of momentary strength, repetition by repetition, by a set of intensive exercise. More than 30 years ago, I heard Arthur Jones discuss inroad in the following manner.

Let's say on a seated biceps-curl machine, you can do 10 repetitions with 80 pounds of resistance. In spite of your best effort, you cannot do an 11th repetition. You're done. You're spent. Why did you fail? Did your biceps strength go from something above 80 pounds down to zero?

The answer is no. Here's why: If you're a typical trainee, your repetition-by-repetition strength drops an average of 2 percent per repetition. On repetition 1, you are 100 pounds strong—and 100 pounds of strength easily curls 80 pounds of resistance. On repetition 2, you are 98 pounds strong, and 98 pounds lifts 80 pounds, and so on. On repetition 10, you are approximately

80 pounds strong—and 80 pounds of strength, with a little body English or cheating on your part—is barely able, with a supreme effort, to curl 80 pounds on the machine. On repetition 11, you are 78 pounds strong—and 78 pounds of strength will not curl 80 pounds of resistance.

Continuing that example, from one set of 10 repetitions, you've made a 22 percent inroad into your starting level of strength for your biceps.

According to Jones and much Nautilus research, the most consistent level of muscular growth occurs when a trainee makes an inroad of 15 to 25 percent on the majority of exercise sets.

From my own strength-training history, I knew that my strength was fairly typical. In fact, my average inroad on most exercises paralleled the 2 percent, repetition-by-repetition, inroad described above. With most of my exercises, I could expect to perform approximately 10 repetitions with 80 percent of the resistance I could do one time maximally. Using a repetition style of 2 seconds on the positive and 4 seconds on the negative, 10 repetitions required approximately 60 seconds for me to perform—and then I failed on the 11th repetition.

The X-Force Example

In Chapter 9, I discussed how my first experience on two X-Force machines revealed to me the negative-accentuated advantage. It's worth another look.

In my private gym in Florida, I had a leg curl machine and a biceps machine that were almost identical to the X-Force versions, with one major exception. The X-Force machines had a tilting weight stack that provided 40 percent more resistance on the negative.

In my trial test, I knew exactly the amount of resistance that I handled in Florida a week earlier. So in Stockholm, I loaded the X-Force leg curl and biceps machines with the same resistance—that is, the same resistance in the positive but that provided me with 40 percent more in the negative. Then I performed as many repetitions as possible in good form (2 seconds on the positive and 4 seconds on the negative). Following are my results:

My machines in Florida, repetitions: leg curl, 10; biceps, 10

X-Force machines in Sweden, repetitions: leg curl, 7; biceps, 7

The time it took me to perform 10 repetitions on each machine in Florida was 60 seconds, and the time it took me to do 7 repetitions in Sweden was 42 seconds. That demonstrated that, with X-Force, I achieved almost the same inroad as I did at home, 21 percent versus 22 percent, in 42 seconds, as opposed to 60 seconds. Thus, the X-Force leg curl and biceps machines, for me, were approximately 50 percent more demanding per repetition (3 percent inroad versus 2 percent) and required 30 percent less time to failure (42 seconds versus 60 seconds).

Degree of inroad per repetition and time required to failure revealed to me that X-Force, compared with conventional equipment, provides more efficient inroads. I believe that something similar comes into action with my 30-30-30 style of negative-accentuated training.

Time Under Load

Since you don't have access to an X-Force machine, you can use my 30 seconds negative, 30 seconds positive, 30 seconds negative method to achieve similar results. Yes, 30-30-30 is slightly different in that it's the time under load that's a salient factor, not the increased resistance. But the time under load with the negative phase is twice as long as the positive phase.

When you really get into 30-30-30, and the resistance is ideal, that last 30-second negative feels as though the resistance is much heavier than it actually is. That heavy feeling on the last negative is what you want eventually on all your negative-accentuated exercises.

Today I know that 30-30-30—compared with earlier guidelines—is a much better method, and it produces high-quality muscle-growth stimulation. And a great deal of that credit should go to it for making a deeper inroad into a trainee's momentary strength.

Why not go for 30-30-30?

JOE WALKER

BEFORE & AFTER

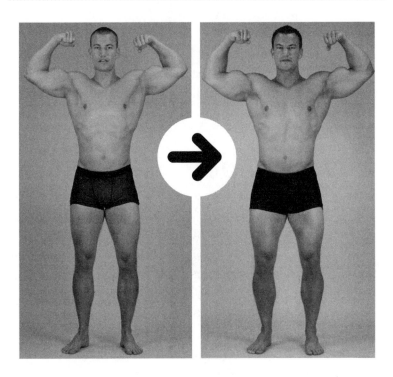

AGE 26, HEIGHT 5'9"

BEFORE BODY WEIGHT

177
POUNDS

AFTER BODY WEIGHT

194.38
POUNDS

AFTER 6 WEEKS*

17.38
POUNDS OF MUSCLE GAIN

2
INCHES ADDED ON ARMS

3.125
INCHES ADDED ON THIGHS

* On muscle-building program only

CHAPTER 13

The Mechanics of Muscle

Intensity + Control + Brevity + Rest = Growth

IF you examine the history of the barbell and its connection to muscle building, you'll learn that it was only about a hundred years ago that people thought that anyone who exercised with a barbell would become muscle-bound and clumsy. Anyone who wanted to use barbells was considered dumb, obsessed, and self-centered.

Today those misconceptions have changed. In the past 2 decades, scientists have taken muscle quite seriously as a marker of good health. Muscle building has come out of the closet.

Here's the current view of how a muscle grows, plus some basic details on body fat.

Muscle Hypertrophy

Muscular growth takes place at the microscopic, cellular level. The basic cells are called sarcomeres. Inside each sarcomere are strings of movement molecules called myosin, which, with tiny cross bridges, connect to a thin protein filament called actin. Myosin, actin, and their interactions—along with the hormone enhancements discussed in Chapter 4—determine the quality and quantity of muscular growth.

The key interaction must occur as a result of muscular-system overload that causes the right amount of microtears to the myosin and actin strings. When the strain on the muscle is focused and intense from controlled negatives, the movement mechanisms pull apart and tear slightly. This exposes frayed myosin and actin strands, which have the ability to attract other growth elements. With appropriate hormone coordination, adequate rest, and nutrients, these units and elements are rewoven into thicker, stronger filaments with new branches.

The units of myosin and actin increase, which causes an expansion in the size of the individual sarcomeres. Because the number of sarcomeres is set at birth, these basic units increase their size for muscular growth to occur.

The Negative Connection and Soreness

A good negative-accentuated workout produces muscle soreness—a lot of it. This condition, called delayed-onset muscle soreness (DOMS), occurs from 18 to 24 hours after an intense workout. The peak soreness may not fully set in for another 24 to 48 hours. DOMS is caused by localized damage to the muscle fibers and the involved myosin and actin tissues.

You'll recall from the chapter on the physics of negative muscle action that the chemical bonds in the lengthening process are extremely stable. But when they are stretched correctly, the subsequent chemistry contributes to the soreness, repair, and growth.

What many trainees fail to realize is that a certain amount of muscle soreness probably benefits muscle development. Once the body perceives

FROM FAT TO MUSCLE: WHAT IT LOOKS LIKE

MANY PEOPLE DO NOT UNDERSTAND HOW body parts change from the loss of fat and the gain of muscle. The example below will help.

Turn to page 93 and look at the before-and-after photos of Jeanenne Darden. Jeanenne lost 29.5 pounds of fat and built 6 pounds of muscle. Her overall body fat dropped from 32 percent to 17 percent. Her before left thigh measured 25 inches and her after measurement was 22 inches, which was a loss of 3 inches.

If we took a magnetic resonance imaging of a cross section of her left thigh, before and after, it might resemble the following drawings:

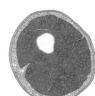

LEFT THIGH CROSS SECTION

Before
Circumference:
25 inches

After
Circumference:
22 inches

Before
Percentages:

Skin	8
Bone	7
Fat	50
Muscle	35

After
Percentages:

Skin	7
Bone	8
Fat	35
Muscle	50

The cross sections are composed of the outer skin, middle bone (white), fat cells (light gray), and muscle cells (dark gray). In the before cross section, excessive fat not only accumulates in thick layers directly under the skin, but it also formed within and around the thigh muscles.

Notice that the amount of fat and the amount of muscle drastically changed. In fact, there was a reversal: The thigh fat shrank from 50 to 35 percent, and the thigh muscle expanded from 35 to 50 percent. The area of the second cross section is 23 percent smaller than the first one.

If you go back and examine the photos of Jeanenne, you'll see that the muscularity and overall shape of her thighs is much better in the after photo than the before.

Interestingly, of the 24 women from Gainesville who were involved with Group 2, 50 percent achieved the same approximate results as Jeanenne's. But they did so in half the time—in 12 weeks, as opposed to Jeanenne's 24 weeks.

damage, immune cells migrate to the damaged tissue to remove cellular waste to help maintain the fiber's overall structure. The body then produces signaling molecules that activate the release of various growth factors. So muscle soreness and its localized inflammation lead to a growth response that eventually strengthens the tissue to withstand future muscle damage.

Look at the negative connection in this manner: Negative-accentuated exercise, properly performed, is the best way to produce DOMS. And muscle soreness means you've engaged fully in the muscle-growth process. Consider it positive feedback on negative-accentuated training. Within a couple of weeks of starting this type of training, you'll actually look forward to the way your body feels after an intense workout.

Out with the Pill, In with the Chill

Stay away from taking anti-inflammatory drugs—such as aspirin, ibuprofen (Advil and Motrin), and naproxen (Aleve)—in an attempt to reduce your soreness. Using these drugs can deter the full saturation of the muscle-growth chemistry that is pervading your system. On the other hand, taking a cold plunge after your workout, or even the day after, helps all the healing and overcompensation processes.

In other words: Out with the pill, in with the chill.

Don't Overtrain

Many of my negative-accentuated trainees in Gainesville had, and still have, a difficult time grasping what I'm about to explain. In fact, it took me many years to completely understand the following concept:

> → Any more exercise than the precise amount required for optimal results is not merely wasted effort, it is counterproductive. Compensation precedes overcompensation.

→ Recovery always comes before growth.

→ Recovery and growth both require time. When you train too long or don't rest enough between workouts to allow for full recovery, muscle growth will not occur.

Important: The amount of training you do isn't as critical as how you do that training. You must constantly strive to execute your exercises under control and with perfect form *and* keep your negative-accentuated sessions as brief as reasonably possible.

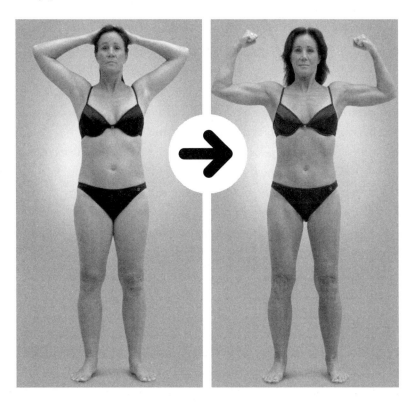

My wife, Jeanenne Darden, 52, assisted me in my negative-training applications.
At a starting body weight of 170 pounds, she lost 29.5 pounds of fat and built 6 pounds of muscle over 6 months.

Before I get into the chapters related to negative-training science, it's time to take a hard look at body fat, the various types, and how to measure it.

The Facts about Body Fat

I learned about the basics of body fat in 1969 at Florida State University from an old-school nutrition professor named Harold E. Schendel, PhD, who kept the fundamentals simple and to the point. Here's how Schendel would have handled questions about body fat.

Q: Exactly what is body fat?

A: *Chemically speaking, body fat is composed of 6 percent proteins, 79 percent lipids, and 15 percent water. Because of the high concentration of lipids, a pound of fat contains 3,500 calories, or about six times the calories of an equal amount of muscle tissue.*

Seen under a microscope, fat tissue looks like a bubble bath. The globules are grouped together with stringy intercellular glue and streaked with narrow filaments of connective tissue, blood vessels, and nerves. This network of fat cells is designed to provide a living inner tube, with minimum stress both to the skin on the outside that encloses it and the organs on the inside that it encloses.

Q: Are there different types of body fat?

A: *Yes, there are several ways to classify body fat. The one that makes the best sense to me divides fat into three types:*

- *Subcutaneous fat lies in layers directly under the skin.*
- *Depot fat is inherited and is deposited in certain areas of the body.*
- *Essential fat cushions and protects the many vital organs.*

Approximately 50 percent of human fat is subcutaneous, 40 percent is depot, and 10 percent is essential. Women tend to have a greater percentage of depot and essential fat than do men. When you lose fat, this fat comes primarily from your subcutaneous and depot sites, but not from the essential areas.

Q: What is the function of fat in the human body?

A: *The primary function of body fat is the long-term storage of fuel. Almost from the beginning of life on earth, fat has had a biological role to play as fuel for moving organisms.*

*Locusts and monarch butterflies prepare for long-distance migra-
tions by preflight feeding and fat depositing that can last for several
days. Before migrating, birds may fatten themselves by 25 percent
in a week. Several species of fish—notably, salmon and sharks—are
recognized for their lipid reserves that provide energy for their long-
distance swims.*

*Except for camels, higher forms of vertebrates tend to store fat less
locally. Fat in humans is distributed all over the body. But in spreading
out under the skin, fat seems to have taken on new functions that may
not have been intended in the evolutionary process. With a girdle of fat
under the skin and around the internal organs, insulation and even heat
production may be added to fat's primary use as an energy storage
depot.*

NEGATIVE TRAINING BURNS FAT

A COMMON MISCONCEPTION AMONG FITNESS-MINDED PEOPLE. Is that
to shed body fat, you must do aerobics. Doing aerobics, it is thought, burns fat
as fuel, while strength training utilizes carbohydrate energy.

What's not commonly recognized is that it really doesn't matter what
type of fuel your body is using. The bottom line is that it requires calories.
More than any other single factor in fat loss, calories count: dietary calories, exercise calories, and metabolic-rate calories. That's why during
negative-accentuated exercise, even though the body relies largely on carbohydrates for energy production, you still lose fat. Those carbohydrates
expended during exercise are replaced by foods eaten, and fat stores are
mobilized to supply energy needs created by the deficit from your exercise
performance, dietary restrictions, and elevated metabolism.

You will make better use of your time by building muscle, because your
muscles will burn extra calories while at rest the next day. That is the
advantage of negative-accentuated training.

Q: *How do I determine how much fat I have in my body?*

A: *Sure, you can see and feel the rolls of fat around your waistline. But how do you put a percentage on the amount of fat you have? Conventional height-weight charts are of minimal help, since they don't measure fat. Scientific methods that are meaningful include calculations based on x-rays, ultrasound waves, underwater weighing, electrical impedance, and skin-fold thickness. Most of these techniques require special equipment and expertise and can be time-consuming and expensive.*

I've had good success using a Lange Skinfold Caliper to measure the thickness of folds of skin and fat in various areas of the body. The method I recommend for taking skin-folds, and in turn calculating the percentage of body fat, comes from work done by the late Michael L. Pollock, PhD, and is cited in the Bibliography. You can probably schedule a skin-fold/fat assessment at your local YMCA, fitness center, or university exercise science department.

Also, in Chapter 24, you'll find out how to estimate your percent body fat by using what's called a pinch test.

....

POP QUIZ

OKAY, HERE'S MY POP QUIZ FROM a favorite lecture of Harold Schendel, PhD. The answer is not in this chapter, but it's somewhere in this book. You have 10 minutes to answer this question:

When you apply diet and exercise to lose fat from your body, where does the lost fat go?

A practical understanding of the correct answer to this question can center you firmly on the road to being lean for the rest of your life.

AEROBICS VS. STRENGTH TRAINING

Which Improves a Woman's Physical Appearance More?

HUNDREDS OF BOOKS HAVE BEEN PUBLISHED on the physical-appearance benefits of building your muscles by lifting weights or through strength training. Unfortunately, many of them are turnoffs for most women, who continue to prefer aerobics.

Edward Jackowski, the author of *Hold It! You're Exercising Wrong*, interviewed 1,000 women who were enthusiastically involved with aerobics. During the interview, he asked each one, "How many women, including yourself, do you know who have ever vastly improved their bodies by taking aerobics classes?"

Each one of them had the same response: "Zero." Not one woman had lost a significant amount of fat or built much muscle from aerobics. Yet most of these women kept returning day after day and week after week in the hope that something would happen. They twisted, they turned, they stepped, they swayed, and they sweat—but nothing much happened.

Why? The women received poor results because the exercise movements were lacking in intensity. They were not hard enough or progressive enough to produce growth stimulation. High-intensity effort is necessary for body-part improvements.

"Do not take any aerobics classes," Jackowski concluded, "with the expectation that you're actually going to change your body—because you won't. Take them because you enjoy exercising with others. Take them for fun."

I agree with Jackowski's findings. Even under the best conditions—such as with body-pump classes that use light barbells—the repetitions are far too many to be an efficient way to lose fat or build muscle. Anything less than the best conditions produces few results.

The negative-accentuated program, with its deeper inroad, makes you leaner, stronger, and firmer. You'll see and feel results after your very first workout. After only nine workouts, or 6 weeks' worth of the program, the average woman will have, at least, an extra 4 pounds of solid muscle on her body.

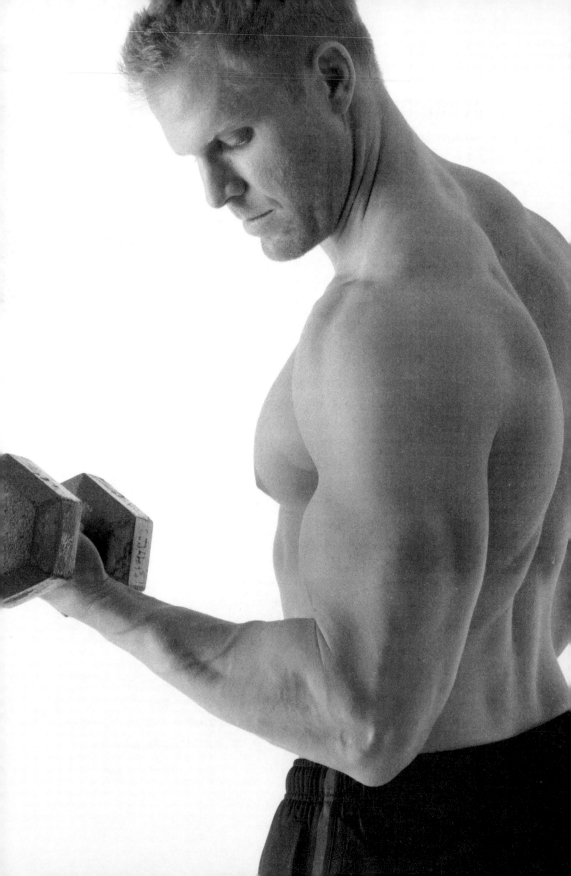

PART IV

Negative-Accentuated Principles and Exercises

CANDACE SPENCER
BEFORE & AFTER

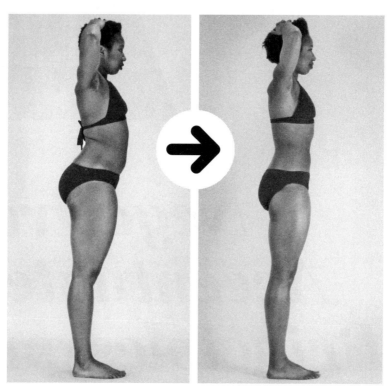

AGE: 21, HEIGHT: 5'5"

BEFORE BODY WEIGHT

154.6
POUNDS

AFTER BODY WEIGHT

130.6
POUNDS

AFTER 12 WEEKS

28.27
POUNDS OF FAT LOSS

10
INCHES OFF HIPS AND WAIST

4.27
POUNDS OF MUSCLE GAIN

CHAPTER

14

Precise Negatives

Mastering intensity, progression, and form

TO get the most out of negative-accentuated exercise, you have to train with great intensity, keep moving forward, and practice proper form. Understanding each of these concepts will help you execute them with precision and success.

Intensity

On a machine exercise, such as the chest press, you normally perform a repetition smoothly with a count of 2 seconds positive and 2 seconds negative. With a repetition scheme of 8 to 12 and stopping when you cannot do another repetition, you might be able to complete 12 repetitions in 48 seconds. This is a *normal* style of training.

The key to a normal style of high-intensity training is to never stop a set until you are sure you cannot perform another positive half repetition.

If you took 80 percent of that resistance and wanted to slow the rep to a creep, you could do a half repetition positively (the pushing) in 20 seconds and another half repetition negatively (the lowering) in 20 seconds. That would be one repetition, 40 seconds, performed in an *extremely slow style.*

If you wanted to accentuate the negative or lowering, which we do in this book, then the preferred way is to take 80 percent of the resistance that you normally handle for 8 to 12 repetitions. Have an assistant help you on the first positive half repetition, then take at least 20 seconds on the negative, 20 seconds on the positive without help, and a final 20 seconds on the negative. (Note: If you can do another half repetition positive, then the resistance was probably too light.)

Performed properly, this 20-second negative, 20-second positive, and 20-second negative (60 seconds total) equals 40 seconds of negative work and 20 seconds of positive work—or twice as much emphasis on the negative as the positive. This style of training is called *negative accentuated.*

Whether doing the normal, extremely slow, or negative-accentuated style of training, the key to getting maximum results is to select a heavy enough resistance that you are barely able to finish, in good form, the last few seconds of the positive phase and the last few seconds of the negative phase.

Those last few seconds of both phases, or half repetitions, are painful and produce a burning sensation in the muscles involved. But you must learn to work efficiently through the burn and continue for a while longer. Pushing yourself to do this right is the key to success.

Progression

In normal exercise, progression means that with each workout, you should try to add another repetition, additional resistance, or both. In extremely slow and negative-accentuated style, instead of adding repetitions, *time under load* is the progressive factor.

With negative-accentuated-style exercise, after you can do 20-20-20, the next progression is 25-25-25, then 30-30-30. When you can successfully perform a 30-second negative, a 30-second positive, and a 30-second negative, that's the signal to increase the resistance by approximately 5 to 10 percent at the next workout. That will reduce the time under load to approximately 20-20-20. Then you continue the progression as before.

With normal lifting, the increase in resistance is 2 to 5 percent. But in the negative-accentuated style, the increase is greater, 5 to 10 percent. Negative training allows for greater gains of strength, thus the greater jumps in resistance.

Form

How properly you perform the exercise matters as much as intensity and progression. Although the exact form that I recommend for each exercise in the Body Fat Breakthrough program will be described in another chapter, some generalities apply to all the movements:

→ **Keep momentum low.** It's to your advantage to use momentum—bouncing or throwing—during a weight-lifting contest, in which it's all about hefting as much as possible any way you can. But this book does not promote weight lifting for contests. Excessive momentum is cheating in this book. It subtracts from your goal of exhausting your muscles as thoroughly as possible. Momentum makes the exercise easier, when the goal is to make it harder. Lower and lift smoothly, with no jerks and sudden movements. Pay attention to the turnarounds at the bottom and top, and keep them controlled.

→ **Move slowly, smoothly.** The negative-accentuated style keeps the speed of movement necessarily slow. Just make sure the movement is smooth and not a series of stops and starts.

→ **Use as much range of movement as comfortably possible.** On single-joint exercises, pause in the contracted position but not in the stretched position. On multiple-joint pulling exercises, pause in the contracted position but not in the stretched position. On multiple-joint pushing exercises, stop short of locking your knees and elbows, and do not pause in the flexed position. More details will be covered on each of the categories of exercises in Chapter 16.

Bringing It All Together

Since the early 1960s, I've trained tens of thousands of fitness-minded people. But I've trained only one man who exceeded my expectations during the very first workout. That's Joe Cirulli, the founder and owner of Gainesville Health & Fitness.

I had known Joe for more than 3 decades, but I never took a close look at his training. And I never personally trained him.

On April 9, 2012, I pushed Joe Cirulli through a tough X-Force workout. Cirulli was 59 at the time, 5 feet 9 inches tall, and weighed 201.5 pounds.

My goal was to preset the 10 selected X-Force machines and move him quickly from machine to machine, with no rest periods. The workout that Cirulli performed was similar to the machine routine listed in Chapter 26 for weeks 5 and 6.

Cirulli didn't break. He went from machine to machine with no rest. He didn't pause for a drink of water. He hardly blinked.

Yes, he stumbled a little after the X-Force leg press machine, but that was all. He walked away after the last exercise telling me that he relished the pain and wanted me to make it harder next Monday.

HOW TO BREATHE DURING NEGATIVE-ACCENTUATED EXERCISE

THERE'S A NATURAL TENDENCY TO HOLD your breath when exerting. To hold your breath involves Valsalva—commonly termed *Valsalva maneuver* or *Valsalva technique*. This is a medical term that incorporates a back pressure behind a closed airway. It blocks blood from the extremities going back to the heart and drives blood pressure to high levels.

Do not put a scheme to your breathing. The old weight-lifting advice was "Breathe out as you lift, breathe in as you lower." If you attempt to throttle your breathing in any way, you are engaging in a partial Valsalva.

Practice breathing freely. Gradually, you will learn to breathe without forced and excessive ventilation. This will aid your ability to perform sustained, maximum muscle contractions.

And get this: When I looked at the clock, he had moved through 10 exercises in 11 minutes flat.

It was the most amazing negative-accentuated workout I've ever seen anyone do. My hat goes off to Joe Cirulli of Gainesville Health & Fitness.

Joe, I'm not easily impressed. But you impressed me with that workout.

LEARN FROM JOE CIRULLI

In his April workout, Cirulli did every exercise, with a very heavy resistance, almost perfectly. So I asked him afterward about his intensity and his ability to endure pain. These were his answers:

ED: *Joe, do you do anything special before you get ready to train?*

> **JC:** *Before the workout, I get my mind totally focused. I see myself going through each exercise and giving each repetition of each exercise my absolute best effort.*

ED: *What do you think about when the movement gets really tough?*

> **JC:** *I think that now I'm at the point in the exercise that makes a difference. If I stop, I might as well have stayed at home. If I continue, then I want to give it my best effort—not my almost-best effort but my everything-that-I-have-at-that-moment best effort.*

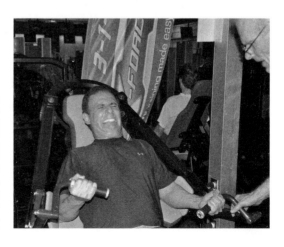

The intensity showed on Joe Cirulli's face as he performed a fifth positive repetition on the X-Force biceps curl machine. Although it looked like Cirulli was unable to move his left arm, he actually finished the positive, did the negative slowly with both arms, and completed a sixth positive and a sixth and final negative repetition. It's important to learn how to pull and push through the pain involved in each exercise and eventually do as many repetitions as possible.

ED: How do you deal with the muscular pain involved in those enduring efforts?

JC: *I totally block out the pain. I sometimes say to myself that it's not real, that it's only imaginary.*

I remember some 30 years ago, I was demonstrating a high-intensity workout during one of your Nautilus training seminars. Jim Flanagan was training me, and 200 people were watching. Halfway through the hardest exercise, the leg press on the compound leg machine, I kept hearing someone in the audience making these loud moaning sounds. Afterward, I asked Jim. "Who was making all that noise while I was trying to focus?" Jim laughed and said, "Joe, the person making all that noise was you." Turns out that I was into the exercise so deeply that I didn't realize I was moaning and groaning. Today I think I do a better job of internalizing the pain.

ED: A lot of trainees can't make it through a hard workout without breaking. How do you keep your composure?

JC: *It goes way back to when I was a kid growing up in upstate New York. When I was 8 years old, I remember being influenced by high school football players who pushed each other during their weight-training workouts. I wanted to do what they did. I wanted to push and be pushed. I wanted more out of myself.*

I remember my early football coach stressing that if you break your focus, your determination, or your desire to win just one time, it will be easier to break the second time and even easier the third time.

I learned early. I never let breaking enter my mind. I do not break.

ED: Joe, that attitude sounds like it's right out of Vince Lombardi's and Don Shula's playbooks.

JC: *It is, and I would have loved playing football for them. But it's also from Norman Vincent Peale, Napoleon Hill, and Earl Nightingale. I review their material with each new year. It never gets old for me.*

Each one of them preached: "Know what you want, stay focused, and continue your step-by-step progression."

When I met Arthur Jones in 1978, I saw a new kind of intensity—both in his training methods and in his commanding style of living. Arthur opened my eyes to new challenges, which I've been working on ever since.

Ellington, you saw Arthur in much the same way I did. He had much influence on you, too.

ED: Yes, you're right. Arthur made a lasting impression on many people. Thank you, Joe, for sharing your experience and wisdom.

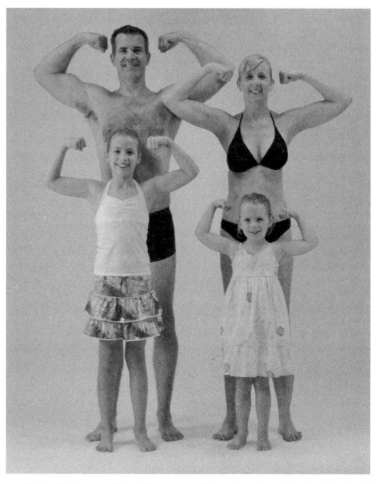

Drs. Ken and Denise Klinker, ages 43 and 40, were one of 10 couples who participated in the Breakthrough program for two, 6-week sessions. Ken lost 31.5 pounds of fat and Denise lost 14.5 pounds. Each added 6 pounds of muscle. They are showing some of that off here with their daughters, Kylie and Chloe.

CHRISTIE WILLIAMS
BEFORE & AFTER

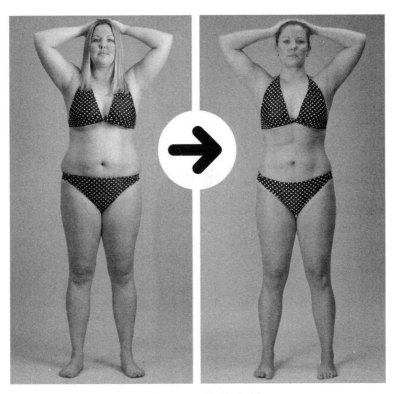

AGE 30, HEIGHT 5'9"

BEFORE BODY WEIGHT

200
POUNDS

AFTER BODY WEIGHT

170
POUNDS

AFTER 18 WEEKS

35.73
POUNDS OF FAT LOSS

8.75
INCHES OFF WAIST

5.73
POUNDS OF MUSCLE GAIN

CHAPTER 15

Duration
and Frequency

How long and how often you should
emphasize the lowering

IF you want to achieve the best-possible results from your negative-accentuated training, you must master the details of workout *duration* and *frequency*.

Duration

Negative-accentuated workouts must be brief. Negative exercise has an effect on the entire body that can be either good or bad. If negative-accentuated work is followed by an adequate period of rest, muscular growth and increase in strength will result. This intensive work, however, must not be overdone.

Many athletes make the mistake of performing far too much exercise using this style. They do too many different movements, too many sets, and too many workouts within a given period of time. When an excess amount of exercise is performed, total recovery between workouts becomes impossible. Negative-accentuated training becomes equally impossible.

You can have brief and infrequent negative-accentuated training or long and frequent low-intensity workouts. But you cannot perform long and frequent periods involving negative-accentuated training. Attempting to do so will produce rapid and large-scale losses in both muscular mass and strength. It may result in total collapse.

When following a fat-loss program, never do more than 10 different exercises in any one training session. The lower body should have 2 or 3 exercises and the upper body, 6, 7, or 8. But avoid going over 10 total. If you push yourself to deliver a supreme effort in each of 8 to 10 exercises, then you'll need only one set!

A negative-accentuated exercise performed in the 30-30-30 style takes 1½ minutes to complete. Allowing 1 minute between exercises, you should be able to complete 10 exercises in just 25 minutes or less. This is one of the key benefits of this style of exercise: It's efficient; you save lots of time.

Frequency

Rest for at least 3 days between negative-accentuated workouts. In fact, 4 days of rest is better in many cases. And 7 days between workouts appears to be even better.

For the Gainesville pilot programs, we divided 6 weeks into three 2-week segments. For weeks 1 and 2, we trained subjects twice a week, on Mondays and Thursdays, and we applied 5 exercises. During weeks 3 and 4, we increased the exercises to 6. During weeks 5 and 6, we increased the exercises to 8—or 10 on some routines—but reduced the frequency to once a week.

Subjects who continued for a second 6-week program—and 80 percent did—were trained only once a week with 8 or 10 negative-accentuated exercises.

Our program, which included reduced-calorie eating for fat loss and twice-a-week training with only 4 or 5 exercises, worked very well. Bringing the small groups of dieters together twice a week gave the individuals confidence in what they were doing. During the last 2 weeks, the small groups of dieters cut back to training and meeting once a week. And again, during the second 6 weeks, the majority of participants preferred once-a-week training.

Supervision

Perhaps you can push yourself to a 100 percent effort occasionally on one or two exercises. Going through an entire routine with 100 percent effort is very difficult to do consistently.

Negative-accentuated exercise is not easy. Properly performed, it is brutally hard, so hard that few people can do it on their own initiative. They need an instructor or training partner to supervise and urge them to utmost exertion.

An example from running should help clarify this concept.

An athlete can run 400 meters in 50 seconds. When he does this, it is a 100 percent effort. His pain during the last 100 meters will be almost

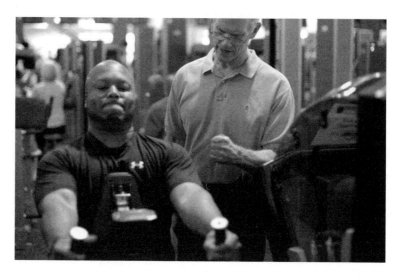

This photo was taken during the first Breakthrough program at Gainesville Health & Fitness.
Here, I'm coaching Jonas Oliver in lowering the last repetition at the ideal speed on the X-Force Lat-Back Row machine. In 6 weeks, Jonas lost 37.19 pounds of fat and built 6.94 pounds of muscle.

unbearable. He rationalizes that if he slows down slightly to run the distance in 55 seconds, then he will probably get 90 percent of the results. If he repeats the 400 meters three times, he falsely reasons, he will accomplish more than by running the track one time with 100 percent effort.

But he will never get the degree of results from running 55-second 400 meters three times that he would by running the track with one supreme effort. It's the 100 percent effort that forces his body to overcompensate and get stronger. *Ninety percent efforts, regardless of the number of times they are repeated, will never approach the results attained by one 100 percent effort.*

The same applies to building strength. If you can do 120 pounds on the chest press in an all-out effort, using the 30-30-30 method, but instead select 110 pounds and perform for the same effort, you have *not* reached your potential.

This is why supervision is all-important. It is doubtful that you can push yourself hard enough, at least during the first 6 weeks. You need a partner to tell you to slow down or speed up, hold your head back, and relax your lower body when you're working your upper body. You must be reminded to eliminate excessive gripping and facial expressions, to keep exerting on that last 30 seconds, and of numerous other details that make each exercise harder and more productive.

Recovery

Adequate recovery time is critical to explosive muscle growth. You need rest to enhance the chemical reactions that repair your tissues and speed up the lay down of new muscle. As I described in Chapter 12, each negative-accentuated exercise makes a deeper-than-normal inroad into the involved muscles' starting level of strength. These combined inroads must be replenished and increased before the next workout is begun.

That's why time and rest are so important. You are much better off getting too much, rather than too little, rest. The primary reason is that your recovery ability does not increase in proportion to your body's ability to get stronger.

Arthur Jones used to graph recovery ability as 50 units and strength potential as 300 units. His graph revealed a 1:6 recovery/strength ratio for most people. In other words, comparing 50 units to 300 units showed that potential recovery ability was disproportionately small, compared with muscular strength potential. Jones's point was that reaching your strength potential requires time: time for rest and time for recovery.

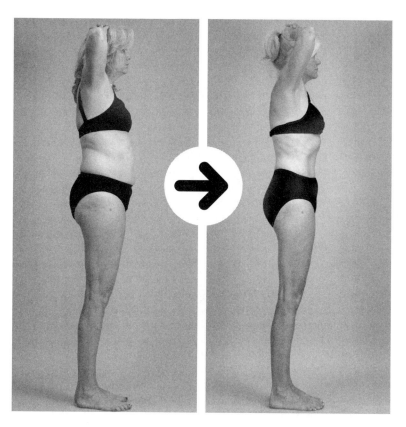

Lynn James, 59, went through the Breakthrough program for two sessions. She lost 22.32 pounds of fat, 5.875 inches off her waist, and built 6.82 pounds of muscle.

DR. BOYD WELSCH
BEFORE & AFTER

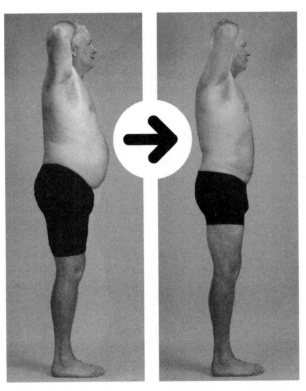

AGE 65, HEIGHT 6'1"

BEFORE BODY WEIGHT

262
POUNDS

AFTER BODY WEIGHT

223.5
POUNDS

AFTER 12 WEEKS

49.27
POUNDS OF FAT LOSS

11.25
INCHES OFF WAIST

10.77
POUNDS OF MUSCLE GAIN

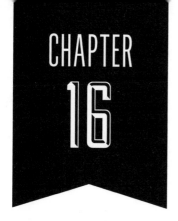

The Negative-Accentuated Exercises

You can use the negative style of resistance training with exercise machines, free weights, or just your own body weight

THIS chapter is full of options for you. It describes in step-by-step detail how to do each exercise in negative fashion. Some of the moves shown here require exercise machines, the kind you'll find in most any gym or health club; others can be done with barbells and dumbbells, or free weights, as they are known. You can even do negatives on your kitchen floor or anywhere you have a little room, using nothing more than your own body weight. The point is, you have an amazing variety of exercises that can be employed for an efficient and effective negative-training workout. But some of the following moves work better than others.

Body weight as the source of resistance has been used for thousands of years as a way to exercise. Today bending, pushing, pulling, and jumping movements using the legs, arms, and torso are widely popular, especially for boot-camp-style fitness classes.

You can certainly use your body weight alone to gain the positive benefits of negatives. But there are caveats. One problem with body-weight movements is that once your strength increases to a certain level, the weight of your body limits the effectiveness of the exercise. In other words, it's harder to progress with body-weight exercises and make them more difficult, because you can't easily make your body instantly heavier. Sure, you can add to your body-weight resistance by wearing a weighted vest; applying raised handles, bars, and padded platforms; elevating the feet; or using just one limb. But for the most part, body-weight exercises have their limits for negative-accentuated training.

Free weights are more versatile for negative training, and better still—for certain exercises—are fitness machines such as Nautilus, Cybex, Hammer, MedX, or Body Solid. Most people don't own these exercise machines and must visit a gym or health club to use them. But with the mix of exercises described on the following pages, you will be able to build a highly effective workout routine no matter what kind of fitness equipment to which you may or may not have access. Get ready to sweat.

Get Ready to Sweat

On the next 48 pages, you'll find my recommended exercises for the negative-accentuated method of lifting, using either the 30-30-30 style or extremely slow repetitions. Each recommended movement is described and illustrated according to the following subheadings:

Preparation: Equipment required, and starting position

Negative: A description of the initial lowering phase of the movement

Positive: A description of the lifting phase of the movement

Finish negative: How to complete the final negative part of the exercise and make it more effective

Tips: Details to improve your results

Note: In most of the photos that follow, image A indicates the starting position of the **negative,** and image B is the starting point of the **positive.**

HOW TO BUILD THE EXERCISES INTO A WORKOUT

Chapter 26 outlines my recommended 6-week workout routines for body-weight exercises and free-weight and machine lifts. I list the exercises you should do each week broken down in 2-week program increments.

You may also choose to create your own workout program. In organizing a negative-accentuated routine, you should select 2 or 3 exercises for your lower body and the remaining ones, usually 4 to 7, for your upper body. One set of 10 negative exercises is the maximum that anyone should perform because they are so physically taxing.

In the training of the 145 people, who composed my test panel at Gainesville Health & Fitness in 2012, the number of exercises per workout varied from a low of 6 to a high of 10. Never was more than one set of 10 exercises performed in any workout by any trainee. Remember, the quality of the exercise is much more important than the quantity. More exercise is usually not better exercise.

To standardize the guidelines, all the body-weight movements will be described in 20-20-20 style: 20 seconds negative, 20 seconds positive, and 20 seconds negative. I do this because it's a great way for anyone to start. After you become familiar with this technique (and build more strength), you will gradually progress to 25-25-25, and, finally, to the ideal 30-second-30-second-30-second negative-positive-negative approach that I've found to be so successful.

PUSHUP

MUSCLES WORKED: PECTORALIS MAJOR, DELTOIDS, AND TRICEPS

PREPARATION

Have a watch or big clock with a second hand in plain sight, or have a spotter help with the counting.

Lie facedown on the floor. Place your hands shoulder-width apart with your thumbs to the inside. Wear rubber-soled shoes and position your feet close together.

Assume the front-leaning position on your toes with your body off the floor and your arms fully extended.

Keep your legs, hips, midsection, and lower back rigid. Viewed from the side, there's a slight S curve in your lower back with your buttocks rising slightly above, but there should be a straight line from your ankles to your head. Your goal is to lower, raise, and lower your body as a unit very slowly, approximately 1 inch with each 5-second count.

NEGATIVE

Hold the top position briefly before you start.

Bend your elbows slightly and lower your body just a little.

Continue to bend and lower inch by inch. You should be approximately halfway down at 10 seconds.

Focus. Relax your face and neck, and don't hold your breath. In fact, breathe often.

Lower another inch and another inch. You should be three-quarters down at 15 seconds.

Keep your chin and hips up. Your chest should barely graze the floor as you smoothly turn around the negative and begin the positive phase.

POSITIVE

Start the positive pushing slowly, 1 inch by 1 inch. Keep your focus and continue breathing. You should be halfway up at 10 seconds. Note: The initial 2 inches from the floor up will be the most difficult part of the pushup. Be prepared to fight through it.

Continue pushing with your arms and chest muscles. Don't let your elbows flare out. Keep them near your torso. You should be three-quarters to the top at 15 seconds.

Check your body and make sure you are still in a reasonably rigid position.

Extend your elbows completely at the 20-second mark. Turn around the movement and immediately begin the finish negative.

FINISH NEGATIVE

Repeat the procedure for the first negative.

Bend your elbows slightly and lower inch by inch.

Try to be halfway down at 10 seconds.

Focus, breathe, and stay rigid.

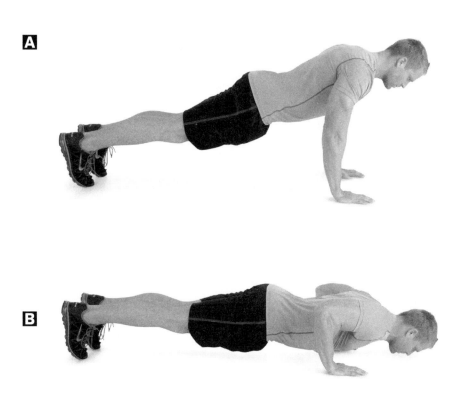

A

B

Give it your all when your chest is 1 inch from the floor and hold for a few more seconds.

Touch your chest to the floor and relax briefly your entire body.

TIPS

Make the negative-accentuated pushup easier or harder.

Easier: *Cut the time to 15-15-15 or even 10-10-10. Do the negative pushup by leaning against a bench that's approximately hip height, which supplies an approximately 45-degree angle between your body and the floor.*

Harder: *Increase the time under load to 25-25-25 and then 30-30-30. Wear a weighted vest, which can be loaded from 10 pounds to as much as 40 pounds. Increase the range of movement of the pushup by using raised handles, such as Perfect Pushup handles, or a couple of hexagonal dumbbells.*

SQUAT

MUSCLES WORKED: HAMSTRINGS, QUADRICEPS, AND GLUTEALS

PREPARATION

Have a watch or big clock with a second hand in plain sight, or have a spotter help with the counting.

Face into a 90-degree corner of a wall. If no corner is available, a sturdy vertical pole, or even the side of a door, will work. If none of these are available, use a flat wall for balance, as shown.

Place your feet a little more than shoulder-width apart, with your toes angled out. Position the fronts of your toes 6 to 12 inches from the bottom of the wall. Try different positions until they feel right.

Lean forward slightly and, with your hands, get the feel of the wall. As you bend your knees, you will be lightly touching the wall to keep your balance.

NEGATIVE

Stand erect in your by-the-wall position.

Start bending your knees slightly, first 1 inch, then 2 inches.

Lower your buttocks smoothly, but keep your lower back slightly arched as you descend. You should be halfway down at 10 seconds.

Breathe as you keep lowering, with your fingers touching the wall if needed.

Go as low as you can without lifting your heels.

Turn the movement fluidly around at 20 seconds and begin the positive phase.

POSITIVE

Push down through your heels, not your toes, as you inch your way up. You should feel an intense contraction in your thighs.

Keep your head and shoulders up and focus on your breathing. You should be nearing the halfway-up position at 10 seconds.

Continue the slow, inch-by-inch ascent. Your hands are helping you balance.

Stand erect at the 20-second mark. Turn around the movement and immediately start the finish negative.

FINISH NEGATIVE

Repeat the slow lowering from the first negative, inch by inch.

Focus, breathe, and keep your core rigid. You should be halfway down at 10 seconds. The hardest part is from halfway down to the bottom.

Exert through your heels and fight the lowering. At 20 seconds, you may want to simply sit on the pillow on the floor.

Relax your entire body briefly and stand.

TIPS

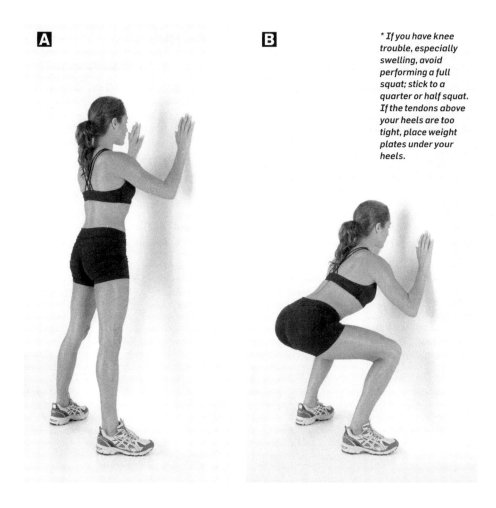

A

B

* If you have knee trouble, especially swelling, avoid performing a full squat; stick to a quarter or half squat. If the tendons above your heels are too tight, place weight plates under your heels.

Push your hips back as you near the bottom, but do not round your lower back. Keep your lower back slightly arched. Problem: People have different bone lengths, levers, and shapes to their calves, thighs, hips, and torsos, which affects their range of motion in squatting. Plus, flexibility issues come into play.

Some people have difficulty squatting below a level where the tops of their thighs are parallel to the floor. Some can almost touch their buttocks to their heels at the bottom. If your ankles are tight and you tend to lift your heels at the bottom, try placing a 1-inch board under your heels for stability.

Make the negative-accentuated squat easier or harder:

Easier: *Cut the time to 15-15-15. Don't go as low on the descent. Use your hands on the wall to help you slow the negative or help you pull up on the positive.*

Harder: *Increase the time under load to 30-30-30. In fact, since your legs are built for endurance, the squat is one of the few lower-body exercises that you could progressively work up to 60-60-60.*

BOTTOM-EMPHASIZED CALF RAISE

MUSCLES WORKED: GASTROCNEMIUS AND SOLEUS

PREPARATION

Because of the short range of motion involved in the calf raise, this exercise is not performed in the negative-accentuated style. Instead, it is worked in a bottom-emphasized manner by dividing the calf raise movement, from a deep stretch to a tiptoed position, in half.

Locate a sturdy 4-inch-thick block of wood or stair step to stand on, with a chair back handy to help you balance.

Wear rubber-soled shoes with treads on the bottom for better grip.

Stand with both feet on the sturdy block of wood, step, or stair. Lean forward slightly. Steady yourself with a chair back or something that will not move (not shown).

Slide your heels off the edge of the block and balance on the balls of both feet.

MOVEMENT

Divide the calf raise in half.
Bottom half: Rise from a deep stretch to halfway up.
Top half: Rise from halfway to high on your big toes.

Do the bottom half for 8 smooth repetitions.

Do the top half for 8 smooth repetitions.

Repeat the bottom half for a final 8 repetitions.

Remember, there are three phases of this exercise: Twice as many bottom-half repetitions, as compared with top-half repetitions, are performed.

Begin with 8 repetitions in each phase. Add a repetition at each workout.

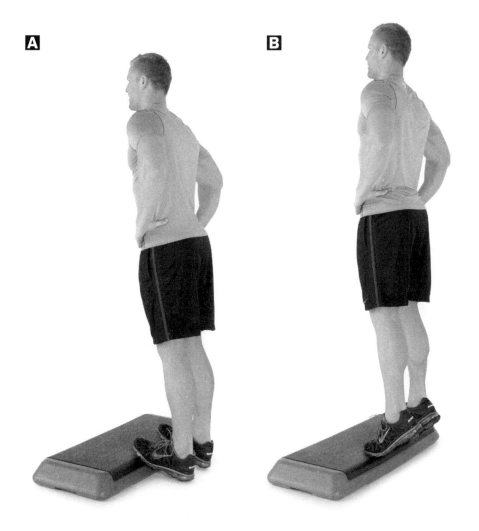

A

B

TIPS

Keep your knees straight during the movement, especially the bottom-half phases. If you do the half repetitions smoothly and slowly, you'll get a deep burn in your back calf muscles—and probably experience some calf soreness over the next several days. Stretch your calves gently for relief, and soak them in cold water for 5 minutes each day. (This man obviously has superb balance. I advise you to place a hand on the back of a chair for stability.)

Make the bottom-emphasized calf raise easier or harder:

Easier: *Shorten the range of movement. Don't go as low on the bottom-emphasized movements.*

Harder: *When you can perform 15 repetitions in each of the three phases, do the exercise by balancing on one leg. This will increase the difficulty of the exercise dramatically.*

CHINUP BETWEEN CHAIR BACKS

MUSCLES WORKED: BICEPS AND LATISSIMUS DORSI

PREPARATION

Have a watch or big clock with a second hand in plain sight, or have a spotter help with the counting.

Place a sturdy bar between the backs of two kitchen chairs. The chair backs should be about 2 feet apart.

Sit on the floor under the bar.

Reach and grasp the bar with an underhand grip, with your hands shoulder-width apart.

Start at the top with your upper chest touching the underside of the bar. Your torso and legs are stiff and at a diagonal. Only your heels are touching the floor.

NEGATIVE

Hold the top position briefly before you start. Again, your body should be stiff, with only your heels touching the floor.

Unbend your elbows slightly and lower your body just a little.

Continue to unbend and lower your body inch by inch. You should be halfway down at 10 seconds.

Lower another inch and another inch. You should be three-quarters down at 15 seconds.

Keep your body stiff. As your shoulders and buttocks near the floor, your elbows should almost be straight. Be ready to turn around the movement at 20 seconds.

POSITIVE

Start pulling up your body slowly, inch by inch.

Keep your focus and breathe. You should be halfway up at 10 seconds and three-quarters up at 15 seconds.

Pull the bar to your upper chest, with your chin well above the bar.

Pause, turn around the movement at 20 seconds, and begin the finish negative.

FINISH NEGATIVE

Repeat the procedure for the first negative.

Lower your body inch by inch.

Try to be halfway down at 10 seconds and three-quarters down at 15 seconds.

Stay rigid and keep breathing.

Sit on the floor at 20 seconds. Relax your grip and remain on the floor for a few seconds longer.

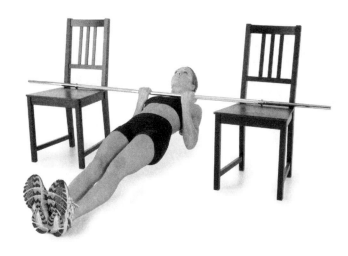

A

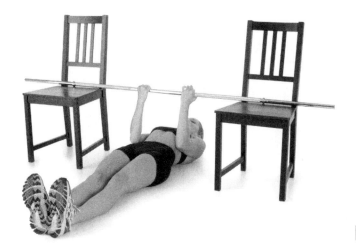

B

The negative-accentuated chinup between chairs may seem extra difficult at first. One tip is to practice keeping your shoulder blades stable and secure throughout the movement. Do not let them spread at the bottom. Once you get the hang of keeping your shoulder blades stable, the pulling will be less demanding and more concentrated.

Women may need to place the bar across the chair bottoms initially, as shown, rather than on the chair backs, to shorten the range of movement and to make the exercise a bit easier. As soon as the shortened range can be performed for 30–30–30, the chairs can be turned and the bar raised so the movement becomes more challenging.

Make the negative-accentuated chinup easier or harder:

Easier: *Reduce the time under load to 15-15-15 or even 10-10-10.*

Harder: *Increase the time to 25-25-25 and then 30-30-30. Wear a weighted vest, which can be loaded from 10 to 40 pounds.*

L-SEAT DIP

MUSCLES WORKED: TRICEPS, PECTORALIS MAJOR, AND DELTOIDS

PREPARATION

Have a watch or big clock with a second hand in plain sight, or have a spotter help with the counting.

Place two sturdy kitchen chairs side by side, approximately $2\frac{1}{2}$ feet apart.

Sit slightly in front of the chairs, so the palms of your hands can be placed on top of the inside chair legs.

Start in the top position with your elbows straight, your heels on the floor in front of you, and your legs straight. As you bend your elbows, your buttocks will drop a little, so that from the side, your torso and legs form an L shape.

NEGATIVE

Hold the top position briefly before you start.

Bend your elbows slightly and lower your body slowly, inch by inch.

Try to be halfway down at 10 seconds and three-quarters down at 15 seconds.

Be ready to turn around the movement at 20 seconds. Do not let your buttocks touch the floor.

POSITIVE

Begin straightening your elbows slowly, inch by inch.

Try to be halfway up at 10 seconds and three-quarters up at 15 seconds.

Pause at 20 seconds in the top position, tighten your triceps, and begin the finish negative.

FINISH NEGATIVE

Repeat the procedure for the first negative.

Bend your elbows slightly and lower your body slowly, inch by inch.

Try to be halfway down at 10 seconds and three-quarters down at 15 seconds.

Pause briefly near the bottom, hold tightly with your triceps, and gradually sit on the floor at 20 seconds.

Remove your hands from the chair and relax briefly on the floor.

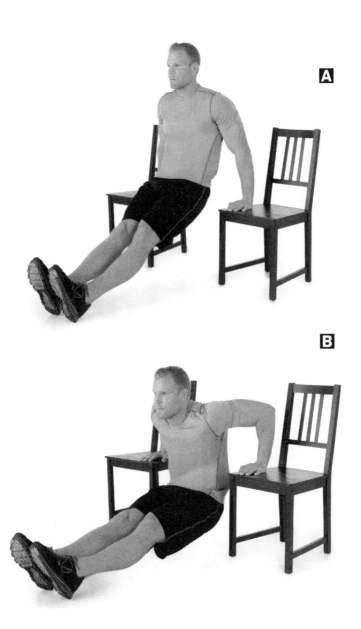

A

B

TIPS

Make sure your hands are in a stable position on the inside legs of the chairs. You don't want the chairs to tip or slide. Do not place the chairs too wide apart. Keep the inside legs slightly wider apart than your shoulders.

Make the negative-accentuated L-seat dip easier or harder:

Easier: *Reduce the time under load to 15-15-15 or even 10-10-10.*

Harder: *Increase the time to 25-25-25 and then 30-30-30. Elevating your feet on the bottom of a third chair makes the movement more difficult.*

SITUP

MUSCLES WORKED: RECTUS ABDOMINIS AND EXTERNAL OBLIQUES

PREPARATION

A BOSU ball is required for this movement. *BOSU* stands for "both sides utilized," but the half ball will be used only with the flat side on the floor and the round side up. If a BOSU ball is not available, you can improvise by using a sofa cushion on top of a couple of thick books.

Note: If this is your first time using a BOSU ball, you should do a few test trials to get the feel and make sure you don't lose your balance. Sitting higher on the ball makes the exercise harder, and sitting lower on the ball makes it easier. Experiment until you get your position just right. Generally, it's best to keep your lower back on the ball through the entire movement.

Have a watch or big clock with a second hand in plain sight, or have a spotter help with the counting.

Sit on the round side of the ball with your knees bent and your feet flat on the floor and apart. The raised ball allows a greater range of movement of the abdominal muscles.

Cup your hands over your ears, and keep your elbows in line with your hands.

Begin with your torso in an upright position.

NEGATIVE

Lower your shoulders and torso slowly, $\frac{1}{2}$ inch by $\frac{1}{2}$ inch.

Try to be halfway down at 10 seconds and three-quarters down at 15 seconds. Keep your head and neck stable.

Arch your back slightly at the bottom and turn around the movement at 20 seconds.

POSITIVE

Curl your shoulders smoothly and move your torso upward, $\frac{1}{2}$ inch by $\frac{1}{2}$ inch.

Relax your face and neck as you move up and forward. You should be halfway up at 10 seconds and three-quarters up at 15 seconds.

Pause briefly in the upright position and turn around the movement.

FINISH NEGATIVE

Repeat the procedure for the first negative.

Try to be halfway down at 10 seconds and at the bottom at 20 seconds.

Remove your hands from your ears and relax at the bottom.

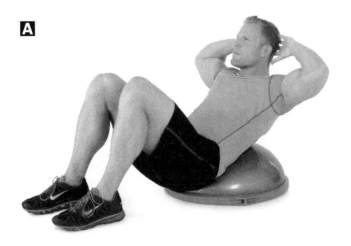

A

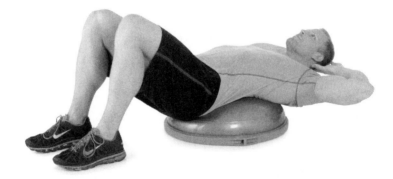

B

TIPS

Do not move your head forward or backward excessively. Do not place your hands behind your head, as this encourages neck strain. Cup your hands over your ears, and don't move your elbows. Keep them even with your ears.

Make the negative-accentuated situp easier or harder:

Easier: *Place your hands across your torso. Reduce the time on the three phases to 15-15-15.*

Harder: *Increase the time under load to 25-25-25 and then 30-30-30. Hold a 10-pound dumbbell or weight plate across your upper chest.*

SIDE CRUNCH

MUSCLES WORKED: EXTERNAL AND INTERNAL OBLIQUES AND RECTUS ABDOMINIS

PREPARATION

Have a watch or big clock with a second hand in plain sight, or have a spotter help with the counting.

A BOSU ball is required for this movement. *BOSU* stands for "both sides utilized," but the half ball will used only be with the flat side on the floor and the round side up. If a BOSU ball is not available, you can improvise by using a sofa cushion on top of a couple of thick books.

Lie on your left side, with your right leg over your left thigh and your feet apart. Test your position on the ball and the placement of your feet until you feel stable. The range of motion in this exercise is short.

Cup your hands over your ears, and keep your elbows in line with your hands.

Begin in a position with your right-side obliques contracted.

NEGATIVE

Hold the top position briefly. Feel the obliques contract.

Lower your head and shoulders slowly, 1/2 inch by 1/2 inch. Keep your hands cupped over your ears.

Uncontract and lengthen your obliques smoothly over 20 seconds to the bottom position.

Stretch the side obliques smoothly and turn around the movement.

POSITIVE

Contract your oblique muscles slowly on your right side as you raise your head and shoulders.

Move through the halfway point at 10 seconds.

Crunch your ribs down toward your right hip at 20 seconds.

Pause and turn around the movement for the last half repetition.

FINISH NEGATIVE

Repeat the procedure for the first negative.

Begin the slow lowering by moving 1/2 inch at a time.

Move past the halfway point at 10 seconds and past the three-quarters point at 15 seconds.

Stay focused and keep your face in a normal position.

Remove your hands from your ears and relax at the bottom.

Stand up, face the other way, and repeat the negative-accentuated side crunch on your right side.

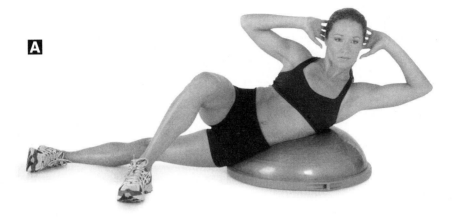

A

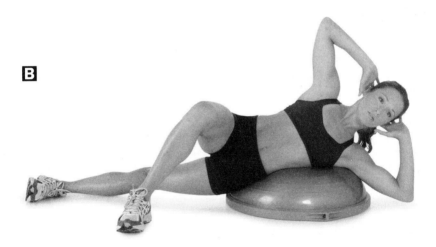

B

Do not let your shoulder drift to your right or left. Stay in the lateral plane on both sides. Alternate the left- and right-side crunch. Do the left side before the right side on your odd-number workouts, and do the right side before the left side on your even-number workouts.

Make the negative-accentuated side crunch easier or harder:

Easier: *Place your hands across your torso. Reduce the time on the three phases to 15-15-15.*

Harder: *Position your hands straight over the top of your head. Hold a 10-pound dumbbell or weight plate over your upper chest.*

BACK RAISE

MUSCLES WORKED: GLUTEALS AND LOWER BACK

PREPARATION

Have a watch or big clock with a second hand in plain sight, or have a spotter help with the counting.

A BOSU ball is required for this movement. *BOSU* stands for "both sides utilized," but the half ball will be used only with the flat side on the floor and the round side up. If a BOSU ball is not available, you can improvise by using a sofa cushion on top of a couple of thick books.

Lie in a prone position on top of the BOSU ball. Your navel should be slightly below the bull's-eye in the center.

Stabilize your lower body by spreading your knees and placing your feet in a reasonably secure position on the floor.

Use your hands and arms to push your torso to a back-arched position, in which your lower back and buttocks muscles are intensely contracted.

Cross your hands over your chest and start the movement.

NEGATIVE

Hold tight in the top position for a few seconds and lower your torso slowly, $\frac{1}{2}$ inch by $\frac{1}{2}$ inch.

Be halfway down in 10 seconds.

Try to touch the floor with the backs of your crossed hands at 20 seconds.

Make the turnaround smoothly.

POSITIVE

Move your torso upward slowly by contracting your gluteal and lower-back muscles.

Keep extending your back and pass the halfway-up point at 10 seconds. Be three-quarters up at 15 seconds.

Pause briefly in the top position and start the finish negative.

FINISH NEGATIVE

Repeat the procedure for the first negative.

Lower slowly in 10 seconds to the halfway position.

Descend the last portion of the repetition in a smooth, focused manner, and touch the floor at 20 seconds.

Relax at the bottom for a few seconds and dismount the BOSU ball.

TIPS

It is not likely that smooth, slow execution of the negative-accentuated back raise would ever involve excessive extension, or hyperextension, of the back or trunk. Yes, the negative-accentuated back raise requires spinal extension and arching of the back or trunk, but the trunk is designed to arch.

If you have a preexisting lower-back problem, it is possible that arching the back may aggravate this condition. But it is also possible that arching the back as described in the negative-accentuated back raise may relieve the problem.

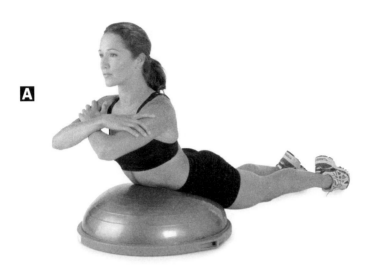

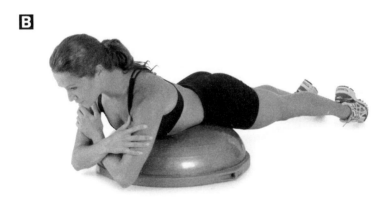

Certainly you need to be cautious and careful in performing any lower-back movement. But remember, arching of the back is normal and should not be an issue with a healthy back.

Make the negative-accentuated back raise easier or harder:

Easier: *Place your hands and arms beside your trunk and hips.*

Harder: *Cup your hands over your ears and keep your elbows wide apart.*

BARBELL BENCH PRESS

MUSCLES WORKED: PECTORALIS MAJOR, DELTOIDS, AND TRICEPS

PREPARATION

Have a watch or big clock with a second hand in plain sight, or have a spotter help with the counting.

Set up a barbell with an appropriate resistance on the support racks of a flat bench.

Lie on your back on the bench.

Grasp the barbell with your hands positioned slightly more than shoulder-width apart.

Straighten your arms and bring the barbell to a supported position above your sternum.

NEGATIVE

Lower the barbell slowly, 1 inch by 1 inch.

Try to be halfway down at 10 seconds and three-quarters down at 15 seconds.

Touch your sternum at 20 seconds but do not rest.

Make a smooth turnaround and begin the positive.

POSITIVE

Press the barbell smoothly, 1 inch by 1 inch.

Be halfway up at 10 seconds and three-quarters up at 15 seconds.

Stay focused and breathe.

Continue pressing deliberately, and make the turnaround at 20 seconds.

FINISH NEGATIVE

Repeat the procedure for the first negative.

Control the negative and lower the bar 1 inch by 1 inch.

Be at the halfway-down point at 10 seconds.

Fight the lowering. Don't let the resistance force the bar down too fast.

Reach the bottom at 20 seconds.

Have the spotter quickly help you get the barbell back to the support racks at the top.

Move off the bench and relax.

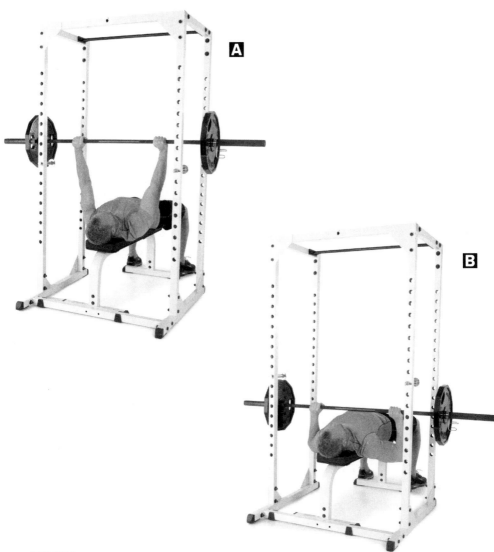

TIPS

This exercise takes some practice. Play it safe, and use only 60 percent of what you'd normally handle for 10 repetitions during your first workout.

Stabilize your starting position by squeezing your shoulder blades together and holding them that way throughout the exercise. Make sure the bar remains directly above your elbows at all times.

Avoid using a wide grip on the bench press. Since the function of your pectoral muscles is to move your upper arms across your torso, spacing your hands wider apart than your shoulders actually shortens your range of motion. Rather than working more of your chest muscles, you're working less of them.

Use a spotter on the negative-accentuated barbell bench press.

BARBELL SQUAT

MUSCLES WORKED: GLUTEUS MAXIMUS, QUADRICEPS, HAMSTRINGS, AND ERECTOR SPINAE

PREPARATION

Have a watch or big clock with a second hand in plain sight, or have a spotter help with the counting.

Place a barbell inside a power rack in the top position on the hooks.

Take two horizontal restraint bars and place them appropriately in the lowest deep-squat position of your range of motion (not shown). These bars protect you from going too low, losing your balance, and possibly injuring yourself.

Load the barbell with the appropriate amount of resistance.

Position the bar behind your neck across your trapezius muscles and hold the bar in place with your hands. If the bar cuts into your skin, pad it lightly by wrapping a towel around the knurl.

Straighten your knees to lift the bar from the hooks and move back one step.

Place your feet shoulder-width apart, toes angled slightly outward. Keep your upper-body muscles rigid and your torso upright during this exercise.

NEGATIVE

Bend your hips and knees slowly, 1 inch by 1 inch.

Descend gradually to the half-squat position in 10 seconds.

Squat a little farther to three-quarters level.

Reach the bottom position, whereby your hamstrings firmly come in contact with your calves, in 20 seconds.

Make the turnaround gradually from negative to positive.

POSITIVE

Lift the barbell slowly and reach the halfway-up position in 10 seconds.

Keep moving inch by inch and stay focused.

Continue the deliberate movement, and try to arrive at the top position at 20 seconds. Do not straighten your knees. Doing so removes tension from the thighs.

Make a smooth turnaround and start the finish negative.

FINISH NEGATIVE

Repeat the procedure for the first negative.

Bend your hips and knees smoothly and slowly.

Hit the halfway-down mark at 10 seconds and the three-quarters mark at 15 seconds.

Keep your focus and continue breathing freely.

Hold the resistance in the deep-squat position, for a final second or two.

Transfer the barbell to the bottom restraint bars or ask two spotters to grab the ends of the bar and rerack the barbell. Sit down on the floor or stagger out of the power rack carefully and relax.

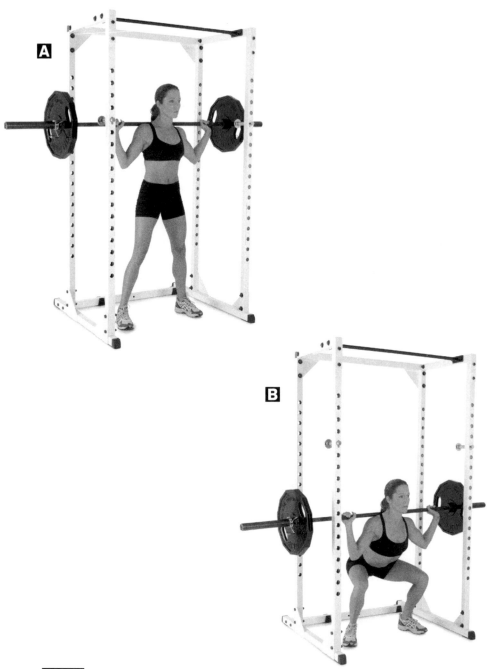

BARBELL CURL

MUSCLES WORKED: BICEPS

PREPARATION

Have a watch or big clock with a second hand in plain sight, or have a spotter help with the counting.

Load a barbell with an appropriate amount of weight, about 75 to 80 percent of what you can normally curl for 10 repetitions.

Take a shoulder-width underhand grip on the barbell. As you stand with the barbell, use some upward momentum and curl the weight efficiently to your shoulders.

Anchor your elbows firmly against your sides and begin the negative.

NEGATIVE

Lower the bar slowly, 1 inch by 1 inch.

Reach the halfway-down position at 10 seconds and three-quarters down at 15 seconds.

Keep your torso erect as you near the bottom.

Turn around the curl at 20 seconds.

POSITIVE

Stabilize your elbows as you curl the bar gradually to the halfway point in 10 seconds.

Keep moving 1 inch by 1 inch.

Pause in the top position at 20 seconds, but do not move your elbows forward. Keep them anchored against the sides of your waist. Doing so allows some of the tension to remain on the biceps.

Turn around the exercise and begin the finish negative.

FINISH NEGATIVE

Start the final descent and progress 1 inch by 1 inch.

Be halfway down at 10 seconds and three-quarters down at 15 seconds.

Keep your elbows anchored firmly against your sides.

Focus on your breathing and don't tense your face.

Stop the curl at 20 seconds.

Place the barbell on the floor, stand, and relax.

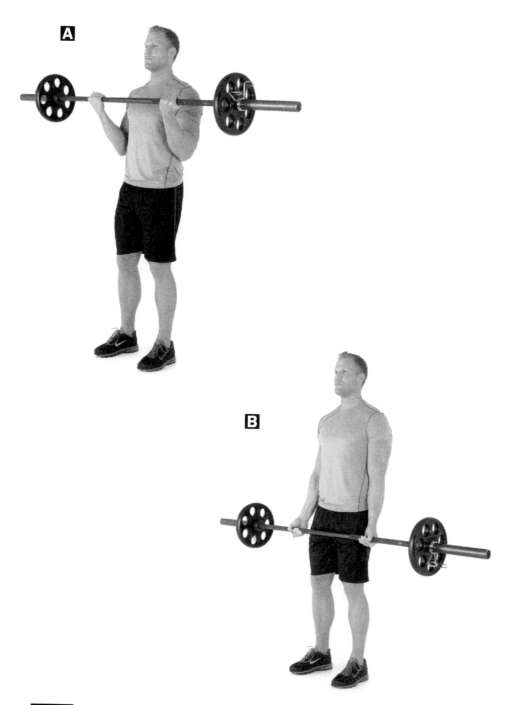

TIPS

Maximize your biceps stimulation by minimizing your body sway. Do not lean forward excessively or lean backward. Do not move your upper arms. Do not move your head. Move only your hands, your forearms, and the barbell.

BARBELL OVERHEAD PRESS

MUSCLES WORKED: DELTOIDS AND TRICEPS

PREPARATION

Note: Even with a lightweight barbell, this is a tough, challenging exercise. Be careful.

Have a watch or big clock with a second hand in plain sight, or have a spotter help with the counting.

Place a barbell on midchest-high hooks in a power rack (not shown).

Load the bar with an appropriate amount of weight.

Grasp the barbell with an overhand grip and position your hands slightly more than shoulder-width apart.

Unhook and lift the barbell, mostly with your legs, and step back with it on your shoulders. Make sure your feet and legs are in a stable position.

Bend your knees slightly and press the barbell overhead. With your elbows completely straight, the barbell should be directly above your shoulders. Ready yourself for the negative phase, as you'll be lowering the bar to your shoulders.

NEGATIVE

Lower the barbell slowly, 1 inch by 1 inch.

Be halfway down at 10 seconds and three-quarters down at 15 seconds.

Focus on your breathing, especially quick exhalations.

Touch your upper chest at 20 seconds and turn around the exercise.

POSITIVE

Press the barbell slowly and smoothly, 1 inch by 1 inch.

Be halfway up at 10 seconds and three-quarters up at 15 seconds.

Lock out your elbows overhead at 20 seconds.

Begin the finish negative.

FINISH NEGATIVE

Repeat the procedure for the first negative.

Guide the barbell down slowly, 1 inch by 1 inch.

Move past the halfway point at 10 seconds and past the three-quarters point at 15 seconds.

Try to control the movement by breathing out at a rapid rate.

Touch your upper chest at 20 seconds.

Move back carefully to the power rack and place the bar securely on the hooks.

Exit the power rack and relax.

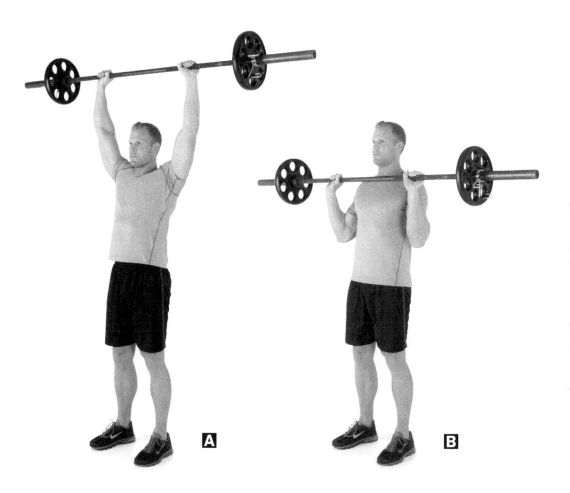

A

B

TIPS

TIPS

Keep your lower back naturally arched during the movements. It may take you several practice sessions to learn the mechanics of the negative-accentuated barbell overhead press, but it will be worth it. This is an excellent exercise for your shoulders and arms, although it can be somewhat challenging for both women and men.

DUMBBELL TRICEPS EXTENSION

MUSCLES WORKED: TRICEPS

PREPARATION

Have a watch or big clock with a second hand in plain sight, or have a spotter help with the counting.

Sit on a bench. Grasp a dumbbell at one end with both hands.

Press the dumbbell overhead.

Pull your elbows in tight and keep them close to your ears throughout the exercise.

NEGATIVE

Bend your elbows and lower the dumbbell slowly, $\frac{1}{2}$ inch by $\frac{1}{2}$ inch.

Reach the halfway-down position at 10 seconds.

Be careful not to move your elbows. Only your forearms and hands should move.

Reach the bottom position at 20 seconds with the dumbbell behind your neck.

Turn around the resistance and begin the positive.

POSITIVE

Straighten your elbows very slowly, $\frac{1}{2}$ inch by $\frac{1}{2}$ inch.

Be halfway up at 10 seconds and completely at the top at 20 seconds.

Pause briefly and begin the finish negative.

FINISH NEGATIVE

Repeat the procedure for the first negative.

Try to be halfway down with the dumbbell at 10 seconds.

Focus and keep good form. Relax your face and breathe.

Reach the bottom at 20 seconds.

Bend forward slightly, lift the dumbbell over one shoulder, and place it on the floor. Or have the spotter grasp the dumbbell from behind your neck.

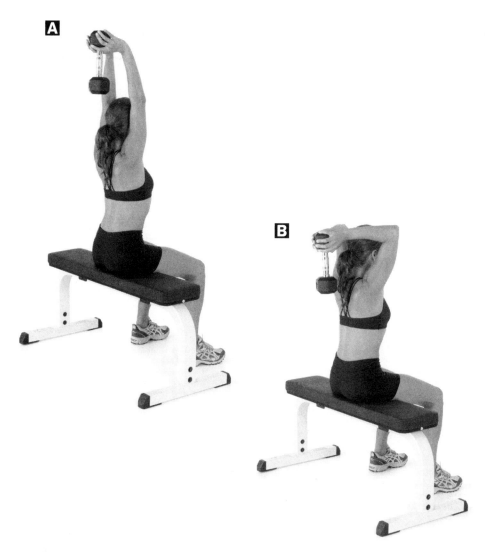

TIPS

Be alert in the bottom position of the negative-accentuated dumbbell triceps extension, as the triceps is stretched across the elbow and the shoulder joints, making it vulnerable to strain. Move in and out of the bottom position very carefully, with no jerks.

BARBELL SHOULDER SHRUG

MUSCLES WORKED: TRAPEZIUS

PREPARATION

Have a watch or big clock with a second hand in plain sight, or have a spotter help with the counting.

This is a short-range movement, so you need to perform the details with precision.

Take an overhand grip on a barbell and stand erect. Your hands should be slightly more than shoulder-width apart and the bar should be touching your thighs.

Shrug your shoulders as high as possible.

Pause and ready yourself for the negative.

NEGATIVE

Lean forward slightly and bend your knees a little. Stay this way through all phases.

Lower the barbell slowly, $\frac{1}{2}$ inch by $\frac{1}{2}$ inch.

Be halfway down at 10 seconds and three-quarters down at 15 seconds.

Sag your shoulders forward and downward as far as comfortably possible at 20 seconds.

Turn around the movement.

POSITIVE

Begin shrugging your shoulders very slowly, $\frac{1}{2}$ inch by $\frac{1}{2}$ inch.

Be halfway up at 10 seconds and three-quarters up at 15 seconds.

Grip the bar intensely as you continue to shrug.

Reach the highest possible position at 20 seconds.

Turn around the movement and get ready for the finish negative.

FINISH NEGATIVE

Repeat the procedure for the first negative.

Lower the barbell slowly, $\frac{1}{2}$ inch by $\frac{1}{2}$ inch.

Be halfway down at 10 seconds and all the way down at 20 seconds.

Pause briefly in the down position.

Place the barbell on the floor, stand, and relax.

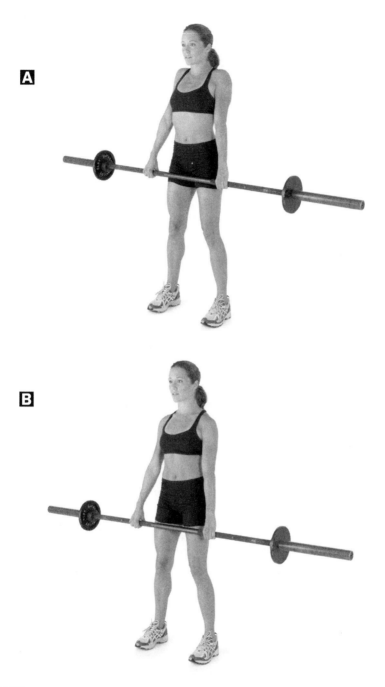

A

B

TIPS

Practice keeping your arms straight and mostly relaxed when shrugging. Bending your arms brings your biceps into action. Keep a slight arch in your back throughout the movement.

SITUP ON DECLINED BOARD

MUSCLES WORKED: RECTUS ABDOMINIS, EXTERNAL OBLIQUES, AND ILIOPSOAS (HIP FLEXORS)

PREPARATION

Have a watch or big clock with a second hand in plain sight, or have a spotter help with the counting.

Locate a situp board assembly that has several levels of raised rungs. Elevating the foot end will increase the difficulty of the negative-accentuated situp.

Sit on the board and anchor your feet appropriately. Anchoring your feet brings more of your hip flexor muscles into action.

Bend your knees and keep them bent through all phases.

Start in the sitting-up position.

Cross your arms over your chest.

NEGATIVE

Lower your torso slowly toward the backboard, $\frac{1}{2}$ inch by $\frac{1}{2}$ inch.

Be halfway down at 10 seconds and three-quarters down at 15 seconds.

Keep your midsection tight as you continue lowering.

Reach the bottom at 20 seconds and turn around the movement.

POSITIVE

Contract your abdominal and hip flexor muscles smoothly and move forward slowly, $\frac{1}{2}$ inch by $\frac{1}{2}$ inch.

Be halfway forward at 10 seconds and three-quarters forward at 15 seconds.

Stay focused.

Round forward at the top at 20 seconds.

Turn around the movement and start the finish negative.

FINISH NEGATIVE

Repeat the procedure for the first negative.

Breathe freely as you start lowering your torso backward.

Move slowly, $\frac{1}{2}$ inch by $\frac{1}{2}$ inch.

Reach the bottom at 20 seconds.

Ease off the board, stand, and relax.

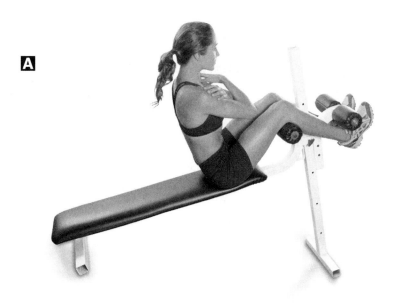

A

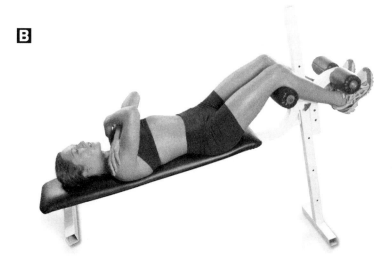

B

TIPS

This exercise requires good form. Practice keeping your face and neck relaxed throughout each phase. Do not reach with your chin on the positive. Keep your knees bent at approximately 45 degrees throughout the exercise. Do not arch your back at the beginning or end of any phase.

Harder: *Make the negative-accentuated situp harder by elevating the foot end of the board, which raises your feet during the exercise. Also, you can increase the difficulty by removing your hands from your torso, cupping your fingers over your ears, and keeping your elbows in line with your head.*

NEGATIVE-ONLY CHINUP

MUSCLES WORKED: BICEPS, LATISSIMUS DORSI, AND HANDS

PREPARATION

The negative-only chinup involves only the negative phase of the movement. The idea is to perform one negative repetition as slowly as possible at the appropriate place in your routine. If you can do a 60-second lowering, which most trainees will have trouble doing, then you'll need to attach additional resistance to a belt around your waist.

While 60 seconds is indeed your goal, both of the negative-only exercises will be described using 30 seconds.

Have a watch or big clock with a second hand in plain sight, or have a spotter help with the counting.

Place a sturdy chair or bench under an overhead chinning bar.

Climb into the top position with your chin above the bar.

Grasp the bar with an underhand grip, with your hands shoulder-width apart.

Remove your feet from the chair or bench and stabilize your body.

NEGATIVE ONLY

Lower your body by unbending your arms slowly, $\frac{1}{2}$ inch by $\frac{1}{2}$ inch.

Be halfway down at 15 seconds.

Lean back slightly and look up. Your knees should be bent and your ankles crossed.

Continue to lower $\frac{1}{2}$ inch by $\frac{1}{2}$ inch until you reach a dead-hang position.

Try to reach the bottom in 30 seconds.

Place your feet back on the chair or bench and exit the chinning bar.

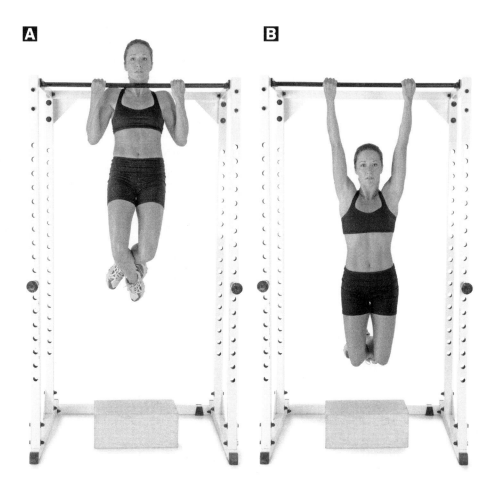

A

B

TIPS

Prevent yourself from moving too fast by trying to stop and actually reverse the movement. You probably won't be able to reverse the movement, but just thinking about doing so will help you slow the descent.

Grip the bar intensely at all times. You do not want your hands to slip. Try to keep your face, jaw, and neck relaxed. Doing so will help you concentrate more on the muscles you're trying to work.

NEGATIVE-ONLY DIP

MUSCLES WORKED: PECTORALIS MAJOR, DELTOIDS, AND TRICEPS

PREPARATION

The negative-only dip involves only the negative phase of the movement. The idea is to perform one negative repetition as slowly as possible, at the appropriate place in your routine. If you can do a 60-second lowering, which most trainees will have trouble doing, then you'll need to attach additional resistance to a belt around your waist.

While 60 seconds is indeed your goal, both of the negative-only exercises will be described using 30 seconds.

Have a watch or big clock with a second hand in plain sight, or have a spotter help with the counting.

Place a sturdy chair or bench between parallel bars. Or use the built-in step or horizontal bar that some dipping bars provide, as shown. Climb to the top position and straighten your arms.

Note: *The bottom finishing position occurs when the backs of your upper arms, when viewed from the side, dip below your elbows. Stop at this point.*

Remove your feet from the chair and stabilize your body.

NEGATIVE ONLY

Lower your body by bending your arms slowly, $1/2$ inch by $1/2$ inch.

Be halfway down at 15 seconds.

Lean forward and keep your elbows tucked close to your body.

Focus, breathe freely, and continue lowering.

Stop the movement at 30 seconds, or when the backs of your upper arms dip below your elbows.

Place your feet back on the chair or attached bars.

Exit the parallel bars and relax.

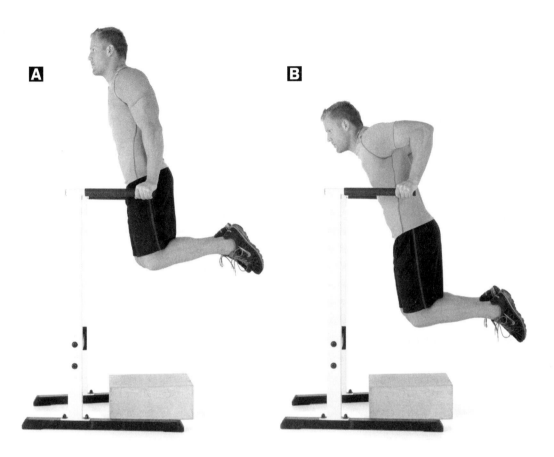

TIPS

Be careful going into the bottom position. You want to feel the stretch more in your chest than your shoulders. Do not go too low. Try to keep your face relaxed.

For these exercises you'll need access to special fitness machines, such as Nautilus, Cybex, Hammer, MedX, or Body Solid.

LEG CURL

MUSCLES WORKED: HAMSTRINGS

PREPARATION

There are several versions of the leg curl machine—prone, seated, and kneeling. The most popular version is performed in a prone position.

Have a watch or big clock with a second hand in plain sight, or have a spotter help with the counting.

Lie facedown on the leg curl machine with your knees on the pad edge closest to the movement arm.

Hook your heels and ankles under the roller pad.

Make sure your knee joints are in line with the axis of rotation of the movement arm.

Grasp the handles on the edge of the machine bench to steady your upper body.

Bend your legs to lift the weight stack. You can do this alone or with the help of a spotter.

NEGATIVE

Hold the contracted position briefly and begin the negative.

Lower slowly, 1 inch by 1 inch.

Try to be halfway down at 10 seconds and three-quarters down at 15 seconds.

Touch the bottom at 20 seconds but do not rest. Turn around the resistance smoothly and start the positive.

POSITIVE

Lift the movement arm slowly, 1 inch by 1 inch. Keep your focus and breathe freely.

Reach the halfway-up position at 10 seconds and three-quarters up at 15 seconds.

Curl your heels smoothly and at 20 seconds try to touch the roller pad to your buttocks. To do so you must arch your back slightly. Do not try to keep your hips down.

Pause briefly in the top position and begin the finish negative.

FINISH NEGATIVE

Ease out of the top position slowly and repeat the procedure for the first negative.

Lower 1 inch by 1 inch to the halfway-down mark at 10 seconds.

Keep your face relaxed, stay focused, and note the three-quarters down mark at 15 seconds.

Resist steadily and reach the bottom at 20 seconds.

Relax your legs, scoot backward, stand, and exit the machine.

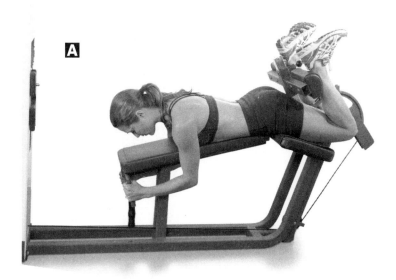

A

B

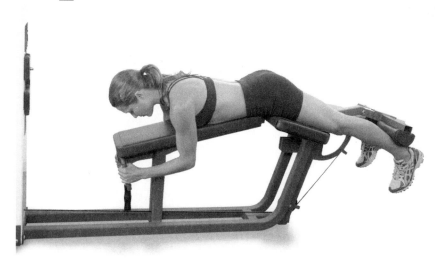

Keep your ankles flexed so that your toes point toward your knees during both the negative and positive phases of the leg curl. This flexion of the ankle stretches your calves and allows for a greater range of motion of the hamstrings.

Place your chin forward during the exercise, as opposed to turning your face to either side.

LEG EXTENSION

MUSCLES WORKED: QUADRICEPS

PREPARATION

Have a watch or big clock with a second hand in plain sight, or have a spotter help with the counting.

Sit in the leg extension machine and place your feet and ankles behind the bottom roller pad.

Align your knee joints with the axis of rotation of the movement arm.

Fasten the seat belt, if one is provided, securely across your hips to keep your buttocks from rising.

Lean back and stabilize your upper body by grasping the handles or sides of the machine. With your spotter's assistance, efficiently lift the movement arm to the top position and pause.

NEGATIVE

Begin the lowering process slowly, 1 inch by 1 inch.

Try to be halfway down at 10 seconds and three-quarters down at 15 seconds.

Keep your focus.

Be at the bottom at 20 seconds and turn around the movement smoothly.

POSITIVE

Start straightening your legs gradually, 1 inch by 1 inch.

Be halfway up at 10 seconds. The next 10 seconds will be the toughest part, so stay in control and concentrate on your quadriceps.

Lean back, not forward, and straighten your knees completely at the 20-second mark.

Pause, turn around the movement smoothly, and ready yourself for the finish negative.

FINISH NEGATIVE

Repeat the procedure for the first negative.

Lower the weight smoothly by bending your legs slowly, 1 inch by 1 inch.

Be halfway down at 10 seconds and three-quarters down at 15 seconds.

Relax your face and emphasize your breathing out.

Fight the last few seconds and set the weight down at 20 seconds.

Be careful as you exit the machine.

TIPS

Keep your feet relaxed during all phases of the leg extension. Do not extend your toes or flex them. Keep them pointing straight ahead in a neutral position. Do not move your head forward or side to side. Practice smooth turnarounds at both ends of the exercise.

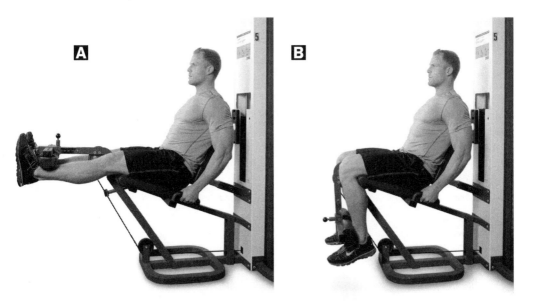

IMPORTANT NOTE

Recently the leg extension has been discussed as a dangerous exercise for two reasons: One, the leg extension tends to stress the anterior cruciate ligament within the knee, which can be problematic for anyone who has suffered ligament injuries to the knee. Two, the leg extension, with the movement arm perpendicular to the lower leg bones, tends to apply shear forces to the knee joint.

As a consequence, some researchers and trainers believe that compression forces from the leg press and the squat are more beneficial to the knee than shear forces from the leg extension.

I've applied the leg extension with thousands of trainees. Plus, I've used it in the rehabilitation of many knee injuries, including anterior cruciate injuries and after surgery. My 40 years of training experience have shown me that almost any strength-training machine or strength-training free-weight exercise—if used incorrectly, which usually means fast and jerky with too much resistance—can cause or lead to an injury. On the other hand, almost any machine or exercise—if applied correctly, such as in the negative-accentuated style described in this book—can be beneficial and a productive way to stimulate muscular size and strength.

If you currently have a knee problem and want to play it safe, the leg extension machine may not be the best option for you. The leg extension remains an important strength-building exercise that offers benefits to the quadriceps that other exercises cannot provide.

LEG PRESS

MUSCLES WORKED: GLUTEALS, QUADRICEPS, AND HAMSTRINGS

PREPARATION

There are many versions of the leg press machine. This one shown involves a diagonal movement footboard.

Have a watch or big clock with a second hand in plain sight, or have a spotter help with the counting.

Sit in the machine with your back against the angled pad and your buttocks on the seat bottom.

Place your feet on the footboard with your heels shoulder-width apart and your toes pointed slightly outward.

Straighten your legs and release the stop bars of the machine (be sure to lock these stop bars at the end of your set to secure the footboard).

Grasp the handles beside the seat, or the edge of the seat, during the exercise.

NEGATIVE

Lower the footboard slowly by bending your hips and knees.

Try to be halfway down at 10 seconds and three-quarters down at 15 seconds.

Turn around the resistance smoothly at 20 seconds. Do not stop and rest at the bottom. Barely touch and start the positive immediately.

POSITIVE

Press the weight and the footboard smoothly, $\frac{1}{2}$ inch by $\frac{1}{2}$ inch. This is the hardest phase of the exercise, and you must learn to move deliberately and steadily out of the turnaround.

Try to pace your movement and be at the halfway-up position at 10 seconds and the three-quarters position at 15 seconds. You'll need to practice working through the muscle burn during this phase.

Reach the top position at 20 seconds, but do not lock your knees. Keep a slight bend in your knees.

Turn around the positive and begin the finish negative.

FINISH NEGATIVE

Focus intensely and remember: You have more strength in the negative than the positive. If you just completed a 20-second positive, you're still strong enough to do a final 20-second negative. Doing so successfully is the most important of these phases.

Lower the footboard very slowly, 1 inch by 1 inch.

Be at the halfway-down position at 10 seconds and three-quarters down at 15 seconds. The hardest portion is the last 5 seconds.

Keep your face relaxed and breathe freely. Don't set the footboard on the stops until 20 seconds are completed.

Have your spotter help you out of the machine or assist you in pressing the resistance back to the top position.

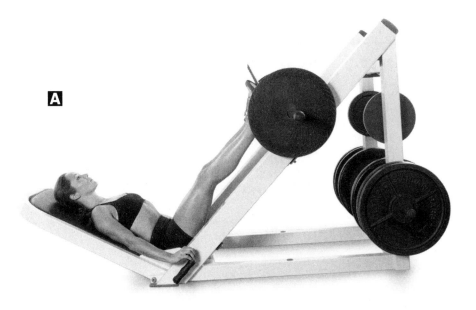

A

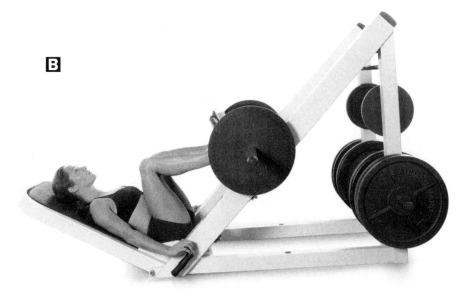

B

The leg press is a very demanding exercise. Work diligently on keeping your movement slow and continuous. Practice keeping your face and neck relaxed.

CHEST PRESS

MUSCLES WORKED: PECTORALIS MAJOR, DELTOIDS, AND TRICEPS

PREPARATION

Have a watch or big clock with a second hand in plain sight, or have a spotter help with the counting.

Adjust the seat bottom on the chest machine so your hands can comfortably grasp the bottom handles of the movement arm.

Sit tall and grasp the handles in your hands. Keep your shoulder blades together throughout the movement.

Straighten your elbows and move the weight stack efficiently to the top position, or get assistance from your spotter.

NEGATIVE

Lower the resistance slowly, 1 inch by 1 inch.

Reach the halfway-down level at 10 seconds and the three-quarters-down point at 15 seconds.

Continue the deliberate lowering until 20 seconds have elapsed.

Turn around the resistance smoothly and begin the positive.

POSITIVE

Move out of the bottom gradually. Press continuously without jerking.

Reach the halfway-up position at 10 seconds.

Continue to the three-quarters level and be almost at the top at 20 seconds.

Turn around the resistance slowly and start the finish negative.

FINISH NEGATIVE

Repeat the procedure for the first negative.

Fight the lowering 1 inch by 1 inch. Stay in control and breathe freely. Keep your face relaxed.

Be halfway down at 10 seconds and completely down at 20 seconds.

Ease off the movement gradually. Remove your hands from the handles and relax.

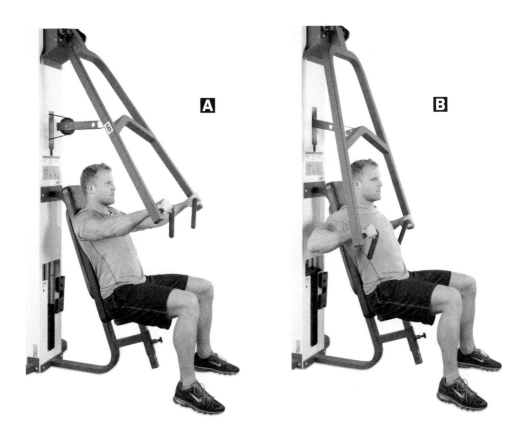

TIPS

Do not move your hips during the positive phase or arch your back excessively. Do not move your feet during either the negative or positive movements. Keep them grounded on the floor.

LAT MACHINE PULLDOWN

MUSCLES WORKED: BICEPS AND LATISSIMUS DORSI

PREPARATION

Have a watch or big clock with a second hand in plain sight, or have a spotter help with the counting.

Grasp the pulldown bar on a lat machine with an underhand, shoulder-width grip and be seated.

Stabilize your lower body properly.

Pull the bar down to your chest efficiently, which lifts the resistance, and ready yourself for the negative.

NEGATIVE

Pause briefly with the bar touching your upper chest. Your elbows should be down and back and holding steady.

Unbend your arms and begin lowering the resistance slowly, 1 inch by 1 inch.

Be halfway down at 10 seconds and three-quarters down at 15 seconds.

Stretch your arms at the top and turn around the bar at 20 seconds.

POSITIVE

Pull slowly, 1 inch by 1 inch, by bending your elbows.

Be halfway up with the resistance at 10 seconds and three-quarters up at 15 seconds.

Complete the pull at 20 seconds. Pause briefly and turn around the movement for the finish negative.

FINISH NEGATIVE

Repeat the procedure for the first negative.

Unbend your elbows and lower the resistance slowly, 1 inch by 1 inch.

Be halfway down at 10 seconds and three-quarters down at 15 seconds.

Stay in control and breathe freely.

Stretch your arms and back at 20 seconds.

Allow the resistance to bottom out on the weight stack, stand, and exit the machine.

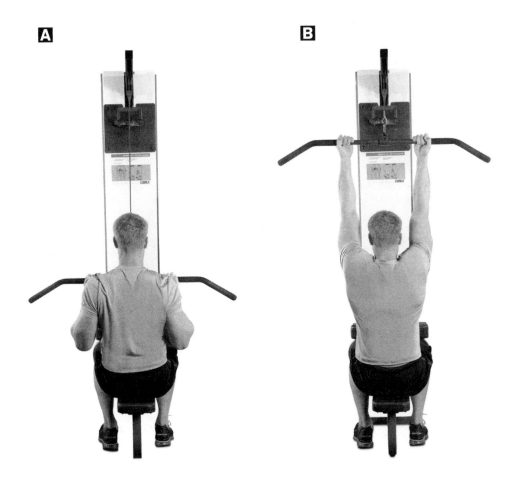

A **B**

Keep your torso upright during the negative and positive phases. Minimize body sway and practice strict form.

ABDOMINAL CRUNCH

MUSCLES WORKED: RECTUS ABDOMINIS AND EXTERNAL OBLIQUES

PREPARATION

Many different types of abdominal machines are manufactured today. I like the ones where the work is performed in an upright, seated position, with a pivot point at the midsection and a movement arm slightly above the shoulders.

Have a watch or big clock with a second hand in plain sight, or have a spotter help with counting.

Adjust the seat bottom so your navel, when you are seated, is parallel to the axis of rotation on the side.

Fasten the seat belt, if one is provided, across your hips and cross your ankles.

Place your elbows on the pads and grasp the handles lightly.

Get to the contracted position efficiently by pulling with your elbows and ready yourself for the negative.

NEGATIVE

Return the movement arm to the top position by releasing your abdominal muscles slowly, $\frac{1}{2}$ inch by $\frac{1}{2}$ inch.

Be halfway back at 10 seconds and three-quarters back at 15 seconds.

Keep your face relaxed and breathe freely. Do not hold your breath.

Be ready to turn around the movement at the stretched, top position.

POSITIVE

Pull with your elbows and begin shortening the distance between your lower ribs and pelvis.

Keep the movement slow, $\frac{1}{2}$ inch by $\frac{1}{2}$ inch.

Reach the halfway-down position at 10 seconds and three-quarters down at 15 seconds.

Continue to breathe.

Pause briefly in the contracted position at 20 seconds.

Turn around the movement and start the finish negative.

FINISH NEGATIVE

Repeat the procedure for the first negative.

Keep your back rounded as you slowly release or lengthen your abdominal muscles.

Move $\frac{1}{2}$ inch at a time smoothly, and try to be halfway back at 10 seconds and three-quarters back at 15 seconds.

Open your eyes and focus on the count.

Arch your back slightly near the top position and allow the weight stack to touch at the count of 20 seconds.

Relax and exit the machine.

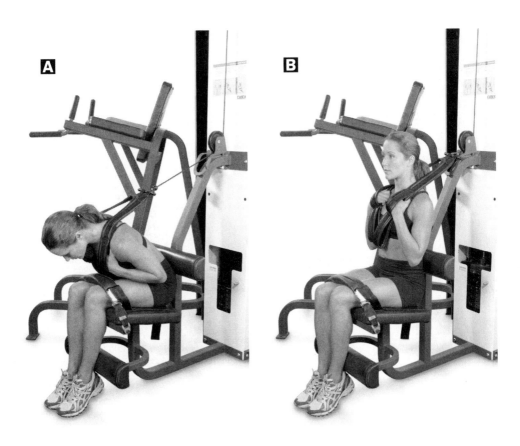

TIPS

Do not jut your chin forward at the start of the positive. Do not try to do a situp on this machine. Try to bring your rib cage closer to your pelvic girdle. Do not pull excessively with your arms. Pull with your midsection muscles.

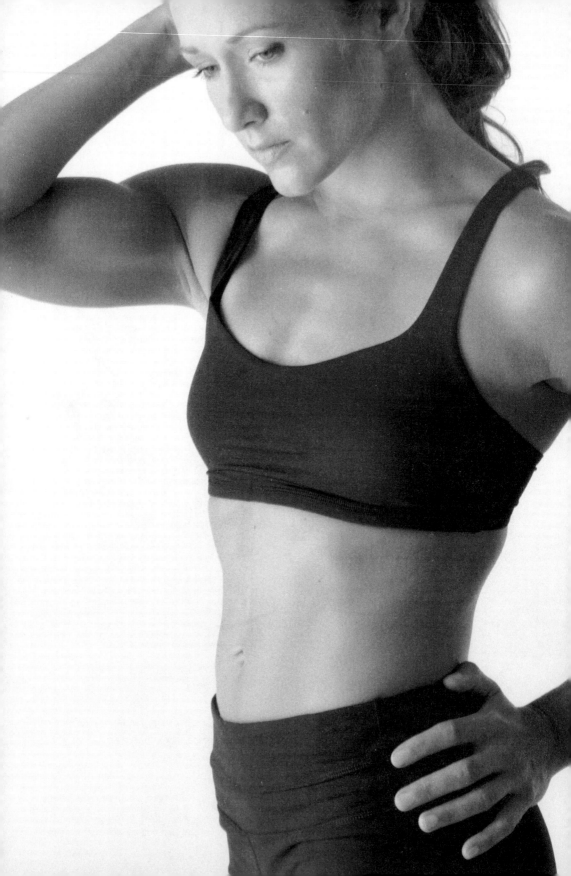

Bombing Your Body Fat

BLAINE HARRIS
BEFORE & AFTER

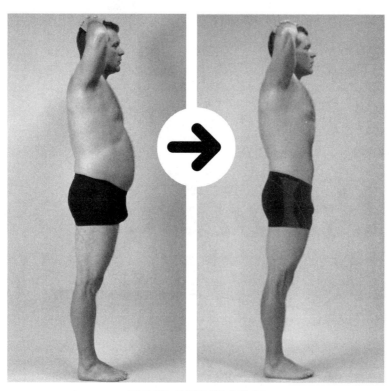

AGE 53, HEIGHT 5'6.5"

BEFORE BODY WEIGHT

168
POUNDS

AFTER BODY WEIGHT

156
POUNDS

AFTER 6 WEEKS

18.36
POUNDS OF FAT LOSS

4.75
INCHES OFF WAIST

6.36
POUNDS OF MUSCLE GAIN

CHAPTER 17

Thermodynamics

The science of heat transfer and fat cell shrinkage

HEAT connects to fat loss, and it also links to fat gain. The relationship is simple, basic, and undeniable—yet it remains largely misunderstood and ignored.

In the science of thermodynamics, body fat is a form of heat. Heat is measured in calories. The relationship is as follows:

Energy = Fat = Heat = Calories = Energy

Albert Einstein and other scientists proved more than 100 years ago that energy cannot be created or destroyed. It can only be transferred. This is known as the first law of thermodynamics. In other words, you can't really lose fat or heat. You can only transfer it.

Judging from all the phony fat-loss schemes that are advertised and the people who buy them—and keep buying them—this principle is difficult to grasp and easily misunderstood. I'll try to explain it in plain English.

One ounce of fat contains 219 calories. Sixteen ounces, or 1 pound, supplies 3,500 calories of heat energy. Remember, a simple heat calorie has measurement and meaning.

When you lose fat, it transfers out of your body as heat in three ways: through your (1) skin, (2) lungs, and (3) urine. Although you lose a small amount of heat through your feces, it is not thought to be significant unless you suffer from diarrhea. Your skin is actually your body's largest organ, and as much as 85 percent of your daily energy emits through it as heat. You lose heat through your skin by radiation, conduction, convection, and evaporation.

Radiation

Heat radiates from the surface of your body. Remember the Stanford University professors' research with black bears discussed in Chapter 5? The palms of our hands are perhaps our most important radiators, followed by the soles of our feet and our faces and heads. About 50 percent of the calories eliminated through your skin each day are lost as radiant heat.

A tall, lean person has a larger body surface area than another person who is of the same weight but shorter and stockier. Because the tall person constantly loses more calories through radiation, he or she can consume more calories per day than the shorter person. Radiation is partially why shorter people tend to get heavier and taller people tend to remain lean.

Almost all of your skin's surface emits calories through radiation. The exceptions are where the opposing surfaces of your skin limit exposure, such as under your arms. But nature has compensated by increasing the number of sweat glands in those areas.

Conduction

Conduction of heat means the transfer of calories through direct contact. For example, when you get into a cool swimming pool or a cold plunge, heat from your body immediately goes into the water. Water is a much better conductor than air, so you can lose more calories in cold water than cold air. Conversely, if you are in a tub of hot water with the temperature higher than your skin, calories will be conducted to your skin's surface.

Various substances have different capabilities to conduct heat. Air, a poor conductor, can be used as an insulator. Much of the insulation in new homes today works by trapping pockets of air between walls. Clothing is generally a poor conductor; thus, it usually insulates and keeps us warm. But we all have experienced the difference between wearing cotton and wearing wool.

One tip concerning conduction that I learned in 1972 from Olympic wrestlers was that shivering burns three times as many calories as sweating. Olympic wrestlers, before their final weigh-ins, are often frantic to lose that last half pound of fat, which will guarantee a lighter weight classification. Shivering, they found, was the best way to accomplish this goal.

Convection

Your skin disposes of another 15 percent of heat by convection. This means that air circulating around your skin helps move heat away from your body. That's why the wind makes you feel cooler when you bicycle or walk. That's why an overhead fan in a workout room can benefit the cooling process as you exercise underneath it. It's also why the wind-chill reading on a winter day is lower than the actual outside temperature.

Evaporation

Your skin perspires constantly, every second of every day and every night. Except when you openly sweat, you are probably not aware of this unnoticeable perspiration. The reason you are not aware is evaporation.

At ordinary room temperature, the moisture vaporized and lost from your skin and your lungs accounts for approximately 25 percent of the calories lost by your body at rest. One-third of the heat lost by evaporation is removed through your lungs, and the other two-thirds from perspiration.

Humidity, as anyone who lives in the South can testify, has a major effect on how efficiently your skin transfers calories. As the humidity increases, your skin loses its ability to cool by evaporation. That's why playing sports and working in a combination of high heat and high humidity can be dangerous. When the humidity is high, your body has to depend primarily on radiation and convection to eliminate calories.

The Exercise Link

The efficiency of your skin's elimination of calories depends on the blood flow through it. Your skin, your body's largest organ, is richly supplied with arteries, capillaries, and veins. As you shrink your subcutaneous fat, the vessels throughout your skin become more prominent.

The blood vessels of your skin enable this large surface area to control removal of calories, which thereby governs your body temperature. Here's where negative-accentuated training makes a strong connection.

There is no better way to condition, revive, and rejuvenate your skin than to work the underlying muscles. With negative-accentuated training, you can isolate and work any part of your body—from the little muscles of your hands and feet to the large muscles of your thighs and chest—which in turn directs blood to those targeted areas. This surging fluid brings nutrients and heat. The rising heat in the muscle must be released through your skin, which then learns to adapt better by becoming a more efficient thermoregulator.

Besides losing fat or heat through your skin, you also transfer it through your lungs and through your urine.

Approximately 10 percent of your daily calorie and heat loss goes through your lungs, which act as a bellows. Inhalation brings in oxygen-rich air, which is vital for energy metabolism. Exhalation carries out oxygen-poor air and the waste product, carbon dioxide.

The remaining 5 percent of your heat calories are lost through urine. In Chapter 20, I'm going to show you how you can significantly increase your urine production—and calorie loss—by drinking more water.

Transition into the Environment

Lastly, when you lose fat, you transfer heat energy out of your body and into the environment. Once in the environment, it is available for use by other living organisms. With each use, heat energy is once again transferred, and the cycle continues endlessly.

Heat energy is everywhere. In basic biology, we learned that the sun is our ultimate source of heat. The key to understanding solar energy, once again, is the transfer concept.

Humans have no way to take in this energy directly. But plants can trap solar energy by using it to combine with carbon dioxide and water. The product of this combination is a hydrated carbon, or carbohydrate. Only plants have the ability to grow by combining energy from the sun with the elements from air, soil, and water. Animals usually get their energy from consuming plants. Humans get energy from eating both plants and animals.

In simple terms, the sun transfers heat to plants, and plants transfer heat to animals. Both plants (through carbohydrates) and animals (through proteins and fats) transfer heat to humans. Humans transfer heat back to the environment, plants, and other animals. All of these transitions have the capacity to change their forms (solid, liquid, and gas) and places of availability.

How to Apply Thermodynamics

Here are some practices related to thermodynamics that may assist you in losing heat calories:

→ Dress cooler and lighter at work.

→ Take off your coat sooner and keep it off longer.

→ Select short sleeves more often.

→ Don't wear a hat.

→ Turn down the thermostat. Sleep cooler.

→ Leave off socks at home or go barefoot more often.

→ Try to remain uncomfortably cool throughout the day and allow your skin's heating mechanism time to adjust.

→ Negative train in a cooler environment, if possible.

→ Wear light, well-ventilated clothing when you exercise.

→ Minimize sweating by eliminating heat buildup.

→ Apply the cold plunge—or a cold pack or cold shower—after workouts.

→ Avoid sauna, steam, and whirlpool baths, as they cause excessive heat accumulation.

→ Wean yourself from electric blankets and flannel sheets in winter.

NICOLE CANNAROZZI
BEFORE & AFTER

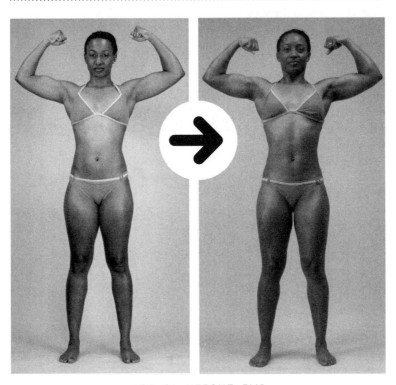

AGE: 31, HEIGHT: 5'4"

BEFORE BODY WEIGHT

134
POUNDS

AFTER BODY WEIGHT

137.2
POUNDS

* On muscle-building program only

AFTER 6 WEEKS*

4.6
POUNDS OF FAT LOSS

1
INCH OFF WAIST

7.8
POUNDS OF MUSCLE GAIN

FAT BOMB #3:
Carbohydrate-Rich Meals

The truth about hydrated carbons and how they help you lose fat

AS a competitive bodybuilder from the years 1962 to 1972, I was persuaded through the muscle magazines of Bob Hoffman and Joe Weider that proteins were "good" and carbohydrates were "bad." (Isn't it funny how that myth is perpetuated today, and not just in bodybuilding circles?)

Harold Schendel, PhD, of the nutrition department at Florida State University, challenged my views, and with the help of several graduate research projects, proved to me that carbohydrates are more important in building muscle and essential to good health than are proteins.

In the last chapter, I talked about heat transfer and the fact that humans have no way to capture the sun's energy directly. Plants, however, can and do by using solar energy to combine carbon dioxide and water. The product of this combination is a hydrated carbon.

Hydrated carbon: Look at the words closely. Now turn it around: *car-bo-hy-drate.* If you're like me, the first time I made that connection, it was like: "How could I have missed that link for so long?"

After pointing that out to me, Schendel was quick to note that carbohydrates are the body's preferred source of energy, and—most important from a bodybuilding point of view—carbohydrates are protein sparing. "Protein sparing" means that adequate carbohydrates allow a moderate amount of proteins to go a long way. By "adequate," Schendel meant that at least 50 percent of daily calories should be carbohydrates. Proteins then can be used directly for repair and building, which is their primary function in human nutrition.

In other words, the body does not have to take proteins, if carbohydrates are limited, and go through a lengthy process to convert them to energy. Hard-core energy, you might say, is the preferred result of carbohydrates, much more so than proteins.

What Schendel proved to me, and what is generally misunderstood by many fitness-minded individuals, is the following:

Carbohydrates should be emphasized, not neglected, by fitness-minded people. The best sources of carbohydrates are vegetables, fruits, beans, and whole grains.

Something else happened that reinforced the importance of carbohydrates.

Birmingham, Alabama, 1973

After the Olympic Games in 1972, I wrote a research report for the *Journal of Home Economics* under the title "Olympic Athletes View Vitamins and Victories." In this report I discussed many of the false beliefs that Olympic athletes had about food and nutrition. One by one, I discussed the reasons why

THE ESSENTIAL NUTRIENTS

WILL THE ABSENCE OF THE CHEMICAL, or substance, in question endanger your health?

Scientists asking that question have determined that an adult requires 45 essential nutrients. If you lack any one of them, sooner or later, your health will suffer.

The 45 nutrients may be divided into the following:

- 19 MINERALS
- 13 VITAMINS
- 9 AMINO ACIDS
- 2 FATTY ACIDS
- GLUCOSE, A SIMPLE CARBOHYDRATE FOR ENERGY (CALORIES)
- WATER

The elements hydrogen, carbon, and nitrogen are not listed, because they are taken for granted as necessary from the environment. Oxygen is also essential, but nutritional science has traditionally limited itself to the study of nutrients that are provided via the digestive system.

vitamin C didn't cure colds, vitamin E didn't increase endurance, high-protein supplements didn't improve muscular size and strength, and low carbohydrates were not the efficient way to lose fat.

As a result of my article, I was invited to speak at the American Dietetic Association's annual meeting, which was held in Birmingham, Alabama, in the spring of 1973. On the same program was Fredrick Stare, MD, PhD, head of Harvard's department of nutrition. Schendel had used one of Dr. Stare's textbooks on nutrition for his nutrition courses at FSU, so I was familiar with his major beliefs. Dr. Stare had been instrumental in the development of the Basic Four Food Groups, which were popularized by the USDA from 1956 to 1979.

After we finished our presentations, Dr. Stare and I discussed how to combat prevalent fat-loss misinformation. Interestingly, the number one best-selling book at that time was *Dr. Atkins' New Diet Revolution,* which was a low-carbohydrate/high-protein eating plan. Dr. Stare had openly denounced the Atkins diet as being nutritionally deficient and dangerous. Much of the initial weight loss that Atkins claimed was fat in fact—according to Dr. Stare—was little more than dehydration from lack of carbohydrates. Dr. Stare noted that there was *no* metabolic advantage, as Atkins claimed, from consuming lots of proteins and fats. The effect was simply one of eating fewer calories because of boredom.

I appreciated the time with Dr. Stare. He was outspoken, witty, and wise. His sage advice to me was: "You'll never go wrong if you always enforce two principles: counting calories and moderation of all foods."

His parting words to me were: "Keep your eye on the basics, my friend, the basics of food and nutrition."

Back to the Basics

From my background in old-school nutrition, my dealings with the recommendations of the USDA, and my experience in working with thousands of fitness-minded people, here are my nutritional guidelines for losing fat:

→ Consume a diet high in complex carbohydrates. Carbohydrates should constitute 50 percent or more of your total daily calories. Eat multiple servings each day of vegetables, fruits, whole grains, and legumes.

→ Maintain a moderate protein intake. Protein should make up about 25 percent of your total daily calories if you are trying to lose fat. If you are trying to maintain your leanness, your protein can go down to 10 to 15 percent and carbohydrates can move up to 60 to 65 percent. Choose low-fat sources of protein.

→ Keep your total fat content at 25 percent of your daily calories. Limit your intake of fat by selecting lean meats, poultry without skin, fish, and low-fat dairy products. In addition, cut back on vegetable oils and butter—or foods made with these—as well as mayonnaise, salad dressings, and fried foods.

→ Avoid too much sugar. Many foods that are high in sugar are also high in fat. Sugar also contributes to tooth decay. (Note: I did not say no white sugar or sucrose. White sugar in small amounts not only improves the taste of many foods but is acceptable on my eating plan.)

→ Don't drink alcohol. Excess alcohol consumption can lead to a variety of health problems. And alcoholic beverages can add many calories to your diet without supplying other nutrients.

→ Drink more water, plain and cold, especially if you are trying to lose fat.

FOOD GROUPINGS

SINCE 1894, THE USDA HAS TRIED to figure out how to depict healthy eating guidelines that will provide all the essential nutrients for an individual. From 1943 to 1956, the guidelines were systematized into the Basic Seven Food Groups.

Fredrick Stare, MD, PhD, of Harvard was instrumental in simplifying the Basic Seven into the Basic Four Food Groups, which I remember well from my third- and fourth-grade health classes. The Basic Four concept was prevalent from 1956 to 1979 and included (1) milk, (2) meat, (3) grain products, and (4) fruits and vegetables. Harold Schendel, PhD, of Florida State University, used the Basic Four in his lectures concerning nutrition and fat loss, and since then, I've applied the Basic Four formula successfully in my fat-loss programs.

From 1979 to 2011, the USDA expanded the Basic Four to five, then six, slightly different groupings and gave them a pyramid shape. Few people actually got the hang of the odd pyramid groupings, so there were 30 years of harsh criticism.

Finally, in 2011, the USDA simplified, condensed, and returned to four food groups (protein, grains, fruits, and vegetables) on a colorful plate, with a bit of dairy on the side. Drs. Stare and Schendel are no doubt smiling.

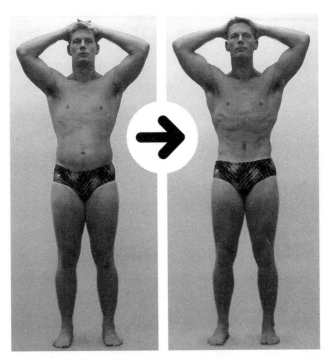

In 2001, Tom Wykle, a professional water-skier, was one of the first athletes in Orlando that I experimented on with a reduced-calorie, carbohydrate-rich diet. Wykle consumed a daily average of 1,900 calories, while performing water-ski shows multiple times each day and strength training three times per week. After 6 weeks, he lost 35.5 pounds of fat, trimmed 5.5 inches off his waist, and built 3.75 pounds of muscle.

The back-to-basics guidelines can still be somewhat general. Over the past 3 decades, I've discovered some interesting behaviors with dieters that, when incorporated, can make the eating process more specific.

→ Dieters can eat the same breakfast and lunch each day for 6 weeks or longer without tiring of it. After 6 weeks, they like a second choice for lunch.

→ Approximately 75 percent of dieters can adapt to a meal-replacement shake for breakfast or lunch.

→ Dieters like a little variety—at least three selections—for dinner.

→ Approximately 90 percent of dieters like the convenience of frozen microwave meals for dinner.

→ Dieters like between-meal snacks.

The next chapter continues with calories per day, meal size, and a simple descent to help you be successful.

FAT BOMB #3

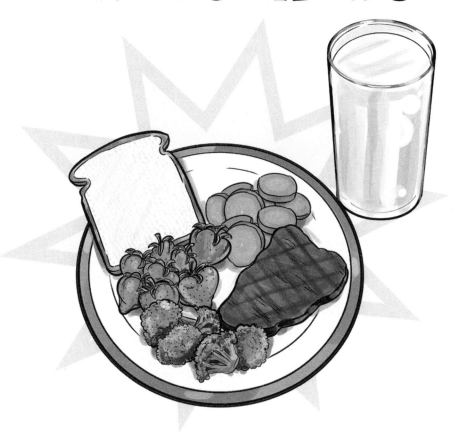

CARBOHYDRATE-RICH MEALS

Consume small meals that are composed of approximately 50 percent of the calories from carbohydrates, 25 percent from fats, and 25 percent from proteins.

CRIS BALDWIN
BEFORE & AFTER

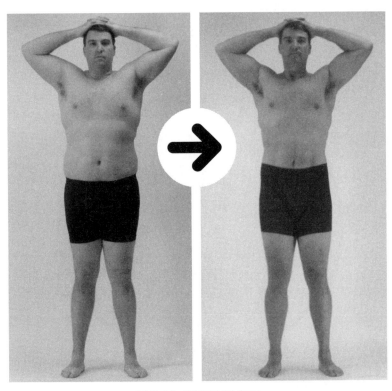

AGE 33, HEIGHT 6'1"

BEFORE BODY WEIGHT

268.8
POUNDS

AFTER BODY WEIGHT

217
POUNDS

AFTER 18 WEEKS

63.74
POUNDS OF FAT LOSS

8.125
INCHES OFF WAIST

11.94
POUNDS OF MUSCLE GAIN

CHAPTER 19

FAT BOMB #4:
Descending Calories

Eat strategically to stay satisfied and melt off flab

"ALL calories have measurement and meaning."
Despite what some authors of popular diet books will tell you, calories count in the weight-loss game. Once a calorie-containing food is consumed, there is no way to weaken, discount, or bypass the effect inside the body.

The laws of thermodynamics are constant, and all things in nature—including human metabolism, muscles, nerves, the heart, and even genes—are governed by thermodynamics.

One gram of carbohydrate and 1 gram of protein each contains 4 calories, while 1 gram of fat contains 9 calories. All these calories from carbohydrates, proteins, and fats count toward either the surplus or deficit of fat metabolism. So the key to manipulating one's weight is to keep from consuming too many. The bottom line is this: To lose fat, you must consume fewer calories than you burn each day.

How Many Calories Per Day

The number of calories you consume in a day should not be too low, or your body may pull nutrients from your muscles and vital organs, which is not what you want. Remember, keeping muscle mass is critical to weight loss and maintenance. The majority of people I've worked with achieve optimum fat-loss results by diligently monitoring their calories. That may sound like sacrifice, but the fact is it works. When combined with negative-accentuated training, it's the technique that will melt off the fat fastest and most efficiently.

Most of the people I've worked with in my weight-loss studies find success on daily calorie levels of 1,800 to 1,200 for men, depending upon body size, and 1,500 to 1,000 for women.

During a 6-week program, I like to descend the calories by 100 every 2 weeks. Such a gradual reduction makes your body more efficient at the fat-burning process.

So I recommend that you try the same, with a descent as follows:

Men: 1,600 to 1,500 to 1,400

Women: 1,400 to 1,300 to 1,200

Meal Size

Fat loss speeds up when you eat small meals. There's a thin line between a small meal and a medium one. I draw that line at 400 calories for women and 500 calories for men.

A large meal of 1,000 calories or more, which is typical in the United States, triggers excessive insulin production. Insulin is your body's most powerful pro-fat hormone. When it's released into your body to deal with a spike in blood sugar triggered by a large meal, it prompts fat storage. Small meals of 400 calories or less, by contrast, bring on small insulin responses that don't encourage fat storage. Thus, it is to your advantage to consume downsized meals. Don't worry. You won't starve. You won't even feel famished if you do it properly. I'll show you how.

DON'T BUY INTO THIS FAD DIET

DURING THE 1970S, SEVERAL POPULAR DIETS promoted the consumption of only 500 calories a day. One pushed a liquid protein supplement, one contained almost all fruit, and one involved a weekly injection of an unusual hormone, human chorionic gonadotropin, or HCG.

Many dieters lost weight on these diets . . . and a few lost their lives.

When you lose weight rapidly, muscle loss can account for as much as 50 percent of your shed weight. Since your heart is a muscle, it can become so small that it will be too weak to pump blood. You can develop an irregular heartbeat and eventually expire from heart failure.

Recently, in January 2013 in Orlando, I saw advertisements concerning a 500-calorie diet and HCG injections, and both the diet and the shots involved medical supervision.

HCG is a hormone produced by the human placenta and extracted from the urine of pregnant women. A British doctor, Albert T. Simeons, introduced the HCG diet in this country more than 60 years ago.

Dr. Simeons claimed that HCG mobilized stored fat for energy. With this stored fat available, he said, a dieter could subsist healthfully on only 500 calories a day. The HCG injections were supposed to suppress appetite while burning the fat off.

Many patients lost weight on this treatment, which is not surprising. Anyone will lose weight on a starvation-level eating plan of only 500 calories a day. But after years of research with HCG, there was absolutely no study that linked HCG to the weight loss. None. Furthermore, the government scientists found no evidence that HCG quieted hunger or helped burn off fat.

Why did people endure the rigors of the HCG diet? (Some are still willing to do so.) Probably because HCG gave them hope in the midst of the desperation that plagues chronic dieters in the United States.

Do not become involved with the HCG diet or any diet that goes below 1,000 calories a day.

Meal Frequency

The trick to consuming less food (calories) without feeling hungry is regular fuel-ups to keep your belly satisfied. The goal is six small, evenly spaced meals a day. This means that no more than 3 hours should elapse between eating episodes. Breakfast, lunch, and dinner are three eating episodes, and there are snacks at midmorning, at midafternoon, and at night. In this book, a snack of 100 to 200 calories qualifies as a small meal.

The size of your meals, the time between your six small meals, and the total number of calories that you consume each day have all been calculated and assembled for your convenience in Chapter 25. But I want to take a moment here to emphasize the importance of the first meal of the day, breakfast—the meal most Americans unfortunately miss—because of its effect on the brain.

Not only are carbohydrates necessary as fuel for your muscles, but they also are vital to your brain. Your brain feeds almost exclusively on glucose, which comes from carbohydrates.

Your blood carries only about 3 minutes' worth of glucose, but your brain needs a continuous supply. Your liver works constantly to keep up with the demand. But your liver can store only approximately 12 hours' worth of glucose.

This is a major reason why you should eat breakfast and include carbohydrates in your midmorning snack. After an overnight fast, your liver is deficient in stored glucose to parcel out for your brain. Breakfast replenishes that store. Even when you're dieting, do not deprive yourself of a high-carbohydrate breakfast and a high-carbohydrate midmorning snack.

Without your high-carbohydrate breakfast and snack, your brain could run short of glucose. If it does, you may feel weak and fatigued or even dizzy. That's not a good way to start your day, and it will hamper your success on the Body Fat Breakthrough program. Eat breakfast!

The methods and programs in this book work. They are based on science, and they are safe. Do they suit everyone? Of course not. But they work for the vast majority of people who fully embrace the program.

If you've had trouble losing fat and keeping it off in the past, I challenge you to understand why calorie restriction is so important to your success and give it a fair trial. You can do it for 6 weeks. I'm certain it will change your body and help you gain control over the power of food.

FAT BOMB #4

1,600 → 1,500 → 1,400

DESCENDING CALORIES

Adhere to a 6-week eating plan that descends the calories
by 100 with each 2-week period.

AUSTIN DEELY
BEFORE & AFTER

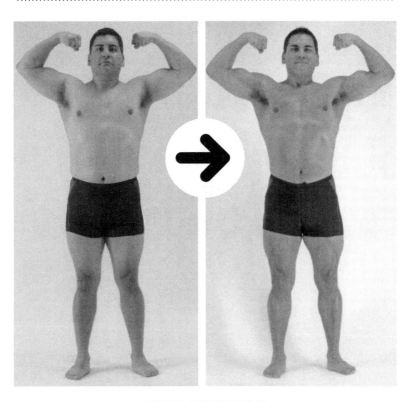

AGE 37, HEIGHT 5'8"

BEFORE BODY WEIGHT

222.5

POUNDS

AFTER BODY WEIGHT

185.5

POUNDS

AFTER 12 WEEKS

43.5

POUNDS OF FAT LOSS

7

INCHES OFF WAIST

6.5

POUNDS OF MUSCLE GAIN

FAT BOMB #5:
Superhydration

Waiter! Water! And make it a double!

THIS chapter should give you the urge to go. That's because it's all about drinking copious amounts of water, more water than you probably have ever consumed before. You need more water because you belong to dehydration nation. Most Americans are walking around dehydrated. We just don't drink enough of the stuff that's so critical to the proper functioning of our bodies. And when we do drink, it's often those sugary beverages that taste great but don't necessarily quench our bodies' thirst for H_2O.

Over the past 25 years, I've written so much about the importance of consuming large amounts of water for fat loss that it's easy for me to take it for granted that everyone knows the truth. Thus, it's a good time to back up and review some of the key reasons why your body thrives on water and how that relates to fat loss.

A Cool Way to Burn

During my initial fat-loss experiments at Gainesville Health & Fitness back in 1985, I started experimenting with having some subjects on my Nautilus Diet consume ice-cold water to curb their hunger. It worked so well that for my next book, I recommended that my new test panel drink a gallon of chilled water per day. It wasn't long before hundreds of women and men at GHF were carrying insulated water bottles to their workouts and wherever else they traveled throughout the day.

It just made sense to me that warming 40°F water inside the body to core temperature, 98.6°F, and then eliminating much of it as warm urine was an excellent way to burn extra calories. (Studies by Michael Boschmann, MD, and other researchers in Germany have proven the validity of this theory.) As as weeks passed, I could measure better results in the group that drank ice-cold water versus the group that drank water that was only slightly chilled.

In 1988 I coined the word *superhydration*, meaning drinking a gallon or more of ice-cold water daily to boost the rate of fat loss.

Your Water Is Showing

The adult human body is made up of 50 to 65 percent water. But not all body components have the same water percentage. Your blood, for example, is 83 percent water, your brain is 75 percent, your muscle is 72 percent, your skin is 71 percent, your bone is 30 percent, and your fat is 15 percent.

As your body experiences dehydration, you feel it first in the systems that contain the most water. For example, you lose your mental alertness and suffer from overall muscular weakness. The last component that dehydration affects is your fat. That's why excessive sweating makes almost no dent whatsoever when you're attempting to reduce your body-fat percentage.

Men have more water in their bodies than women, primarily because men have more muscle mass and less fat than women do. A lean man with a body weight of 180 pounds may have 14 gallons of water in his system. A gallon of water (128 fluid ounces) weighs approximately 8 pounds, so simple multiplication (8 × 14) reveals that 112 pounds of this man's body is water.

FAT BOMB #5

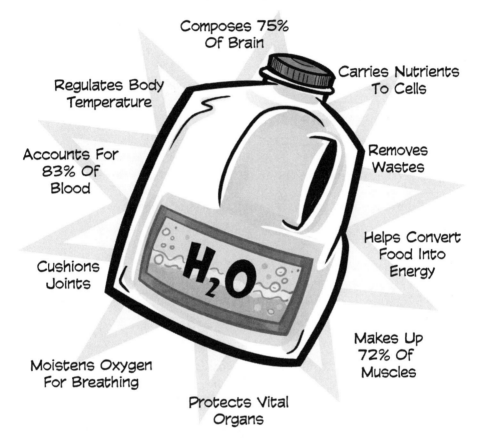

Composes 75% Of Brain

Carries Nutrients To Cells

Regulates Body Temperature

Removes Wastes

Accounts For 83% Of Blood

Helps Convert Food Into Energy

Cushions Joints

H_2O

Makes Up 72% Of Muscles

Moistens Oxygen For Breathing

Protects Vital Organs

SUPERHYDRATION

Drink a gallon (128 ounces) of ice-cold water each day.

You may not think of water as food, but it's the most critical nutrient in your daily life. You can live only a few days without it. Every process in your body requires water. For instance, water:

→ Acts as a solvent for vitamins, minerals, amino acids, and glucose

→ Carries nutrients through the system

→ Makes food digestion possible

→ Lubricates the joints

→ Serves as a shock absorber inside the eyes and spinal cord

→ Maintains body temperature

→ Rids the body of waste products through urine

→ Eliminates heat through the skin, lungs, and urine

→ Keeps the skin supple

→ Assists muscular contraction

How Water Melts Fat

Large amounts of water facilitate the fat-loss process through a number of key body functions.

Kidney-liver function: Your kidneys require abundant water to function properly. If your kidneys do not get enough water, your liver takes over and assumes some of the functions of the kidneys. This diverts your liver from its primary duty—to metabolize stored fat into usable energy.

If your liver is preoccupied with performing the chores of your water-depleted kidneys, it doesn't efficiently convert the stored materials into usable chemicals. Thus, your fat loss stops or at least plateaus. Superhydration accelerates the metabolism of fat.

Appetite control: Lots of water flowing over your tongue keeps your taste buds cleansed of flavors that might otherwise trigger a craving. Furthermore, water keeps your stomach feeling full between meals, which can help take the edge off your appetite.

Urine production: Here's a little-understood fact: As much as 85 percent of your daily heat loss emerges from your skin. Heat emerging from your skin is important because another word for heat is *calories,* and another word for calories is *fat.* That's right: Most of your fat is lost through your skin in the form of heat. Anyway, the remaining 15 percent of that heat loss is divided between warm air coming from your lungs and warm fluid being passed out through urination.

Superhydration can double, triple, or even quadruple your urine production. As a result, you'll be able to eliminate more heat. Remember, inside your body, fat loss means heat loss. So get used to going to the bathroom more frequently than normal. If your urine retains much of its yellow color, you're not drinking enough water.

Cold-water connection: Have you ever wished for a food that supplies negative calories? Let's say such a food exists, and it contains minus 100 calories per serving. Anytime you feel like a piece of chocolate cake or a doughnut, all you have to do to cancel it out is simply follow the sweet with two servings of the negative-calorie food. Presto—plus 200 calories and minus 200 calories yields zero calories. While no negative-calorie food exists in science, ice-cold water has a similar but smaller calorie-canceling effect inside your body.

When you drink chilled water (about 40°F), your system has to heat the fluid to a core body temperature of 98.6°F. This process requires almost 1 calorie to warm each ounce of cold water to body temperature. Thus, an 8-ounce glass of cold water burns approximately 8 calories—7.69, to be exact. Extend that over 16 glasses, 128 ounces, or 1 gallon and you've generated 123 calories of heat energy, which is significant. There's real calorie-burning power in cold water.

A professor of biology from the University of Florida added to my understanding of the cold-water connection when he pointed out that melting ice and a burning candle both require the transfer of heat. They simply modify their forms. The ice changes from solid to liquid, and the candle from solid to gas. Both transfers, or exchanges, involve heat.

Constipation aid: When deprived of water, your system pulls cellular fluid from your lower intestines and bowel, creating hard, dry stools. One of the big roles of water is to flush waste from the body. This is a substantial task during fat metabolism, because waste tends to accumulate quickly. Superhydration tends to make people more regular and consistent with their bowel movements, which is helpful to the overall fat-loss process.

Cold-Water Guidelines

How do you drink a gallon of ice-cold water a day? "With great difficulty," you might reply. Although such a recommendation may sound difficult to follow, in fact, it presents only a few minor problems—such as how, when, and where. Each of these problems can be solved with some intelligent preparation and careful planning.

How: One secret is to not gulp or guzzle the water but to sip it. Get yourself one of those 32-ounce plastic bottles, the kind that has a long straw in the top. I've found that most people can consume water easier with a straw than trying to gulp it down the standard way from a glass. Also, while you're checking out various bottles, select one that is insulated. The insulation will keep your fluid colder for a longer time.

When: Another tip is to spread your water drinking throughout the day. Try to consume 50 percent before noon and the rest before 6 p.m. Drinking most of the water early eliminates the need to get out of bed during the night and visit the bathroom.

Several of our dieters have commented that getting up in the middle of the night to urinate, then going back to bed, leaves them with a feeling of dehydration. If you experience that, it's fine to drink 4 to 8 ounces of water after late-night urination.

Another tip used by patients on an overnight fast before surgery is to suck some crushed ice. Doing so provides a feeling of coolness and moisture without involving an excessive quantity of water.

Where: You sip water everywhere you go during the day because you know how to plan ahead. Once again, you need a 32-ounce insulated plastic bottle. Okay. But what about refilling the bottle, adding the ice, and all the hassle of keeping count of the ounces?

The really motivated people invest in a 2-gallon insulated jug. First thing in the morning, they fill it with ice and water. Then they draw off their initial 32 ounces of fluid into their insulated bottle and start sipping. As soon as the bottle is empty, it's refilled from the jug. When they leave home each day, they carry both the insulated jug and the smaller bottle with them. That way they always have access to chilled water. When they return home in the evening, they carefully wash the jug and the bottle and prepare for the next morning.

Some bottle designs are much easier to work with than others. Usually a larger cap, or a cap at both ends, makes cleaning easier and eliminates the buildup of mildew. Adding a little Clorox is a popular method during cleaning to ensure purity. Keep two bottles on hand so that when one is drying, you can utilize the other.

A great way to keep track of the number of bottles and ounces is to place rubber bands around the middle of the bottle equal to the number of bottles of water you are supposed to drink. Each time you finish 32 ounces, remove a rubber band and put it in your pocket. Four 32-ounce bottles equal 1 gallon, so you'll need to go up and back down with two bands or have four rubber bands total. Four beads on a string would be another system, like an abacus or a rosary.

Additives: There is a difference between plain water and other beverages that contain mostly water. Those mostly water fluids—such as soft drinks, coffee, tea, beer, and fruit juices—contain sugar, flavors, caffeine, and alcohol. Sugar and alcohol add calories. Caffeine—found in coffee, tea, and many soft drinks—stimulates the adrenal glands and acts as a diuretic. Rather than superhydrate the system, caffeine-containing beverages actually dehydrate the body. You should keep such beverages to a minimum.

The only recommended flavoring for water is a twist of lemon or lime. Even so, most of the people who like lemon or lime eventually get to the level where they prefer their water plain.

Tap water or bottled water: In general, the United States has one of the safest water supplies in the world. Chances are high that your community's tap water is fine for drinking. Furthermore, research shows that bottled water is not always higher-quality water than tap water. The decision to consume bottled water or not is usually one of preference.

If you dislike the taste of your tap water, drink your favorite bottled water. Just be sure to check the label carefully for unwanted additives. If you have no problems with the taste of your city's water supply, save some money and consume it.

In fact, many bottled waters are simply city water in plastic bottles. Some safety concerns have been raised about chemicals used for the plastic bottles leaching into the water especially when the plastic heats up during the summer in the Sunbelt states. The other main concern is the presence of chlorine. Chlorine, as pool owners know from the cost, evaporates, so if you obtain a jug of tap water and leave it out on a countertop before pouring it into your container, the chlorine will have evaporated.

Different companies use different plastics for their bottles. Some use glass, although this tends to be more costly and cumbersome because of the extra weight and fragility. There has also been a trend toward stainless steel bottles.

Different Recommendations for Big Men, Small Women

Frequently, trainees in my groups ask me about my blanket recommendation to drink 1 gallon of ice-cold water a day. They want to know if the recommendation should be more for a man weighing 300 pounds and less for a woman weighing 150 pounds.

In 1996, among several fat-loss groups, I tried the following formula: 1 ounce of water for every 2 pounds of body weight. If you weighed 300 pounds (man or woman), you would begin with 150 ounces a day. On the other hand, if you were a 150-pound individual, you would start with 75 ounces. Every 2 weeks, because of your lower body weight, you would recalculate the ounces per day for the next 2 weeks.

This recommendation worked fine in dealing with individuals and with small groups of five people or fewer. But in large groups of 20 to 30, men and women, there tended to be some confusion. And when I looked at the overall fat-loss results between the groups that used the formula versus the ones that applied 1 gallon per day, I found no differences. Everyone had approximately the same fat-loss results.

In the Breakthrough program, I opted for the simplest guideline for both men and women, big and small, young and old: *Drink 1 gallon of ice-cold water a day.*

Too Much of a Good Thing

It's possible to drink too much water, but it's highly unlikely that you would ever do so. In the medical literature, drinking too much water leads to a condition known as hyponatremia. Hyponatremia most often occurs in athletes involved in triathlons and ultramarathons. A few of these athletes consume many gallons of water during the course of these unusually long competitions, and because of the continuous activity, they don't or can't stop to urinate. Thus, they impede their normal fluid-mineral balance and actually become intoxicated with too much water. Such a condition, however, is rare.

I've never observed anything close to intoxication with any of my participants, and some of them have consumed up to 2 gallons of water daily. Of course, they also have no trouble urinating frequently.

Note: Anyone with a kidney disorder or taking diuretics should consult a physician before trying superhydration.

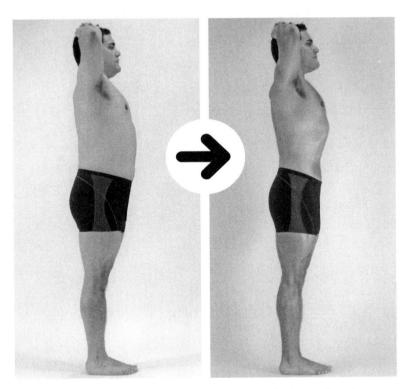

Austin Deely mastered superhydration and applied it productively for 3 months. As a result, he lost 26 pounds of fat during the first 6 weeks and 17.5 pounds during the second 6 weeks—for a total fat loss of 43.5 pounds.

DANA CRASE
BEFORE & AFTER

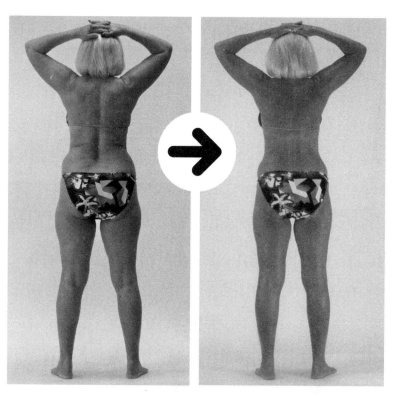

AGE 61, HEIGHT 5'1"

BEFORE BODY WEIGHT

143
POUNDS

AFTER BODY WEIGHT

122
POUNDS

AFTER 18 WEEKS

28.7
POUNDS OF FAT LOSS

6.5
INCHES OFF WAIST

7.7
POUNDS OF MUSCLE GAIN

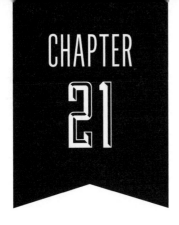

FAT BOMB #6:
After-Dinner Walking

How an evening stroll on a full belly can help increase calorie burn

I receive several e-mail advertisements each week on walking and weight loss. Here are three recent headlines:

"The Easy Way to Walk Off 22½ Pounds in Just 8 Weeks!"

"Walk Yourself Slim"

"Walk Off Your Belly in Just 4 Weeks!"

I'm not a big fan of walking as a productive practice for any component of fitness. Walking does nothing for your muscular strength or joint flexibility. It can produce a limited benefit to your cardiovascular endurance, but not efficiently.

And walking, despite the claims of those misleading headlines in the above advertisements, is not an efficient way to burn calories. So you should cross off walking as a legitimate fat-loss technique—right?

No, no, no. Not so fast!

But you have to stay with me for several minutes as I recover a 1989 study from J. Mark Davis, PhD, and his colleagues at the University of South Carolina's department of exercise science.

Eat a Meal, Walk a Mile

Davis measured and compared seven subjects' calorie burn for 3 hours after completing the following routines: walking only, walking before a meal, and eating a meal before walking. The overall results revealed that the meal-walking routine increased calorie burn among the participants by an average of 30 percent, compared with the other treatments.

The university researchers concluded that going for a walk after you eat triggers what's known as exercise-induced postprandial thermogenesis, and we know now that *thermogenesis* is a welcome word. It simply means "production of extra body heat created by exercising on a full stomach."

Add Water to the Recipe

After a thorough review of the literature on this subject, I was pleased to find that other researchers had studied the effect, and they, too, found that taking a walk after eating a meal can speed up heat production temporarily by as much as 50 percent.

Had anyone studied the thermogenic effect of eating and sipping ice-cold water as a subject walked? I could locate no references. But after discussing the concept with Michael Boschmann, MD, of the Medical Research Center at Humboldt University in Berlin, Germany, he agreed with me that combining all three had to be an even better way of producing heat.

After working with more than 700 trainees—including 145 subjects in 2012—at Gainesville Health & Fitness, I found the following eating-walking-sipping routine to be most effective:

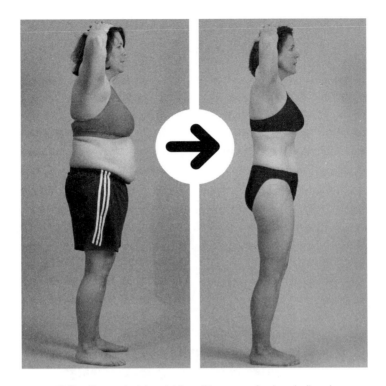

Melissa Norman took her nightly walking very seriously and adhered
to the other Fat Bombs with great consistency—and it paid off. After 12 weeks,
she had lost 39 pounds of fat and dropped 10.625 inches off her waist.

→ Have your evening meal.

→ Begin your walk within 15 minutes after you finish eating.

→ Walk at a leisurely pace for 30 minutes—not 29 nor 31, but exactly
30 minutes. What distance should you walk? A leisurely pace should
cover 1½ miles, which translates to a speed of 3 miles per hour.

→ Carry your insulated water bottle with you. Sip 16 ounces of cold water
as you walk.

→ Wear well-constructed, well-cushioned walking or running shoes. Do
not wear street shoes.

→ Dress in lightweight, comfortable clothes.

→ Walk outdoors, if possible, on level ground. Or you may substitute a bicycle ride for a walk. If the weather is a problem, you may walk indoors or use an exercise bike, treadmill, or elliptical.

→ Do the above each day for 42 consecutive days.

Try my eating-walking-sipping routine each day for the 6-week Body Fat Breakthrough plan and you'll be hooked on a leisurely walk after dinner as a healthy habit for life.

Now take a quick review of the eating-walking-sipping chart and you will see that a 220-pound individual performing the routine for a single day would require 244 calories. Doing the routine every day for 6 weeks, or 42 days, would burn 10,248 calories—almost 3 pounds of body fat.

But get this: Spread that amount over an entire year, and it adds up to more than 25 pounds of fat lost during a fun and relaxing activity that'll do as much for your mind as it will for your body.

CALORIES BURNED FROM EATING-WALKING-SIPPING ROUTINE

BODY WEIGHT IN POUNDS	120	140	160	180	200	220	250	275	300
CALORIES BURNED while walking* 3 mph for 30 minutes	96	111	127	142	159	176	200	219	246
+ 30% FOR MEAL	29	33	38	43	48	53	60	66	74
+ 15 CALORIES for 16 oz cold water	15	15	15	15	15	15	15	15	15
EATING-WALKING-SIPPING ROUTINE: Calories burned	140	159	180	200	222	244	275	300	327

* Walking calculations are from the research of B. E. Ainesworth and colleagues, 2000.

FAT BOMB #6

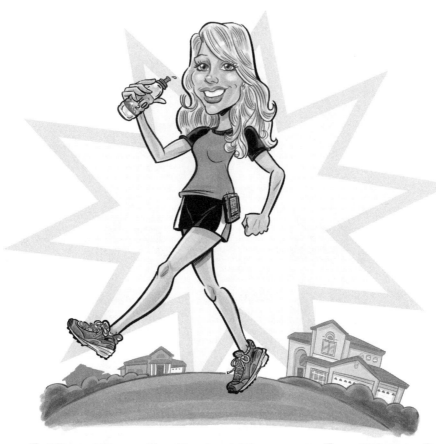

AFTER-DINNER WALKING

Walk daily, after your evening meal, at
a leisurely pace for 30 minutes.

SHANE POOLE
BEFORE & AFTER

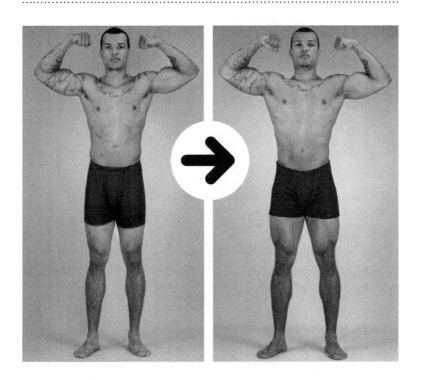

AGE 26, HEIGHT 6'3"

BEFORE BODY WEIGHT

204.5
POUNDS

AFTER BODY WEIGHT

224
POUNDS

AFTER 6 WEEKS*

19.5
POUNDS OF MUSCLE GAIN

1.5
INCHES ADDED ON ARMS

3.75
INCHES ADDED ON THIGHS

* On muscle-building program only

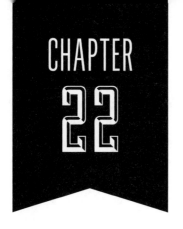

CHAPTER 22

FAT BOMB #7:
Extra Sleep

To build more calorie-burning muscle,
hit the feathers earlier and sleep soundly

"THIS heavy negative exercise makes my body hungry for more sleep," Shane Poole said. "More sleep immediately after the workout and more sleep for at least 3 consecutive nights."

That was unexpected from a big, strong, young man, who from 2006 through 2009 thrived on 5 hours of sleep a night in Iraq, where he was a unit weapons sergeant in the U.S. Army.

When I announced at Gainesville Health & Fitness in March 2012 that I was organizing a group of 15 men who wanted to build significant muscle (and did not need to lose fat), Poole signed up first. (He was by then out of the Army and attending college in Gainesville.) The plan was for me to train each man with negative-accentuated techniques once a week for 6 consecutive weeks. Poole had heard me talking about rapid-rate muscular growth, and he told me that he was going to work harder than anyone else.

He didn't disappoint.

Before his first workout, Poole stood 6 foot 3 inches tall, had a body-fat level of 6.6 percent, and weighed 204.5 pounds. After his number six workout, with no change in his body fat, Poole weighed 224 pounds. That was a gain of 19.5 pounds—19.5 pounds of solid muscle—in 6 weeks.

"I Needed 10 Hours"

"I realized after my first workout, as I was lying on the cool dressing room floor, that I couldn't keep my eyes open," Poole recalled. "Within 30 seconds, I was out—not unconscious but stone-cold asleep. I was out on that hard tile floor for an hour . . . an entire hour.

"I finally got up, spent 5 minutes in the cold plunge, showered, drove home, ate supper, and went to bed—and slept for another 9 hours.

"And I continued to sleep for a good 9 hours each of the next 3 nights—plus an hour nap every afternoon. I couldn't believe it. Most mornings, I'd roll out of bed and look in the mirror and think, 'OMG, I'm bigger.' And I was larger and stronger."

What was happening with Poole's sleep habits—and growth patterns—occurred in at least half of the subjects who were training with similar intensity of effort.

How Much Sleep Is Adequate?

Years ago researchers focused on sleep only as a brain phenomenon, ignoring its effects on other parts of the body. Now they recognize that sleep regulates body temperature, replenishes the immune system, and yields hormones that facilitate fat loss and muscle gain. For a better understanding, let's examine some of the latest facts about sleep.

An infant sleeps 14 hours a day, a healthy teenager averages $9\frac{1}{2}$ hours, and people over 75 years old manage only 6 hours. We sleep less as we age.

These are basic figures. Our modern reality tends to be that our schedules interfere with our sleep patterns. As some comedians like to point out, only civilized people go to bed when they're awake and get up when they're asleep.

Many Americans rely on sleep aids to initiate sleep. Similarly, we rely on alarms to awaken us on time.

We have lost our natural rhythms. The essential one, with some variation during the year because of longer or shorter days, is the circadian rhythm. This is basically the 24-hour, or daily, rhythm.

Before the era of electricity, it wasn't difficult to stay synchronized, because we couldn't see to plow the fields or bring in the harvest, except between dawn and dusk. Our hormonal cycles have remained in this original rhythm rather than adapting—quickly on the evolutionary scale—to the electric light revolution of the past century. The key nighttime hormone is melatonin, and it's easily disrupted by exposure to light, even artificial light.

The latest figures from the National Sleep Foundation (NSF) show that the average adult in the United States gets 6 hours 57 minutes per night during the workweek and 7 hours 31 minutes during weekends. When the numbers are segregated by gender, women tend to fare slightly worse, as they require more time to get themselves, and perhaps other family members, ready every day. This is not adequate sleep, according to the NSF, which recommends that adults get 8 hours of sleep each night.

How to get more sleep: The exercise you'll be getting while following the Body Fat Breakthrough program should help you fall asleep faster and deepen your sleep, but there are other things you can do to improve your sleep habits and reap the benefits of rest.

→ Hit the sack on a regular schedule. Sleep experts say one of the best strategies is maintaining a regular sleep-and-wake schedule. That goes for weekends, too. Staying up later and sleeping in on weekends, your circadian rhythms can affect and reduce the quality of your sleep.

→ Watch out for hidden caffeine. Maybe you're smart enough to avoid the after-dinner espresso, but did you know that colas, chocolate, and even some protein bars contain enough caffeine to activate stress hormones and interfere with sleep, even if you consume them in the afternoon?

→ Stay cool. The National Sleep Foundation recommends keeping your room between 54° and 75°F. A cooler room makes it easier for your core temperature to drop, which is necessary for you to fall asleep.

→ Read a book. This old-school insomniac's cure really works. The repetition of reading lines tires the eyes and helps your brain relax. But avoid reading on your computer. The light from electronic devices suppresses melatonin, the hormone responsible for regulating sleep. Avoid TV, too. The artificial light from television screens can also be interpreted by your brain as daylight, which prevents the release of the sleep-inducing chemical.

Examples of Excessive Stress

There seems to be a definite relationship between lack of sleep and too much stress in a person's life. Getting better-quality sleep tends to help people cope better with stress, and dealing with stress productively tends to allow better sleep.

The classic sign of too much stress is obsessive worry or ruminating about unfinished business that keeps you from falling asleep. When you find yourself trapped in your own thoughts, there are a couple of effective techniques you can try: For an immediate remedy of your overactive mind, get up and walk to another part of the house. (Keep the lights off to avoid triggering your brain to wake up.) Or keep a notepad on your nightstand and write down what's on your mind and resolve to deal with it in the morning. Sometimes that simple act of writing it down can whisk obsessive thoughts from your mind. Another useful mind trick is to simply convince yourself that you have accomplished everything you possibly can for one day and confidently accept that you will complete the job tomorrow.

How does too much stress create a major hurdle to dropping fat? Some of the answer goes back to cortisol, one of your body's primary stress-related hormones.

Cortisol, released by the adrenal gland, prepares the system to take action. Production of the hormone subsides once the endeavor is over. If the stressful event doesn't terminate, however, and continues to perturb you, then some of the hormone remains in your system.

The stereotype is a manager stuck at his desk who flies into a rage with no physical outlet available, except slamming down the phone. It isn't an exaggeration to note that following one crisis too many, managers have sometimes been found slumped over their desks. This was the impetus behind the trend of corporate fitness. A jog, a workout, or a pick-up game of basketball could restore smiles to faces and release built-up tension. Productivity improved, and many more managers reached their full retirement age.

Studies on animals and older people show that long-term exposure to high levels of cortisol can damage brain cells, causing shrinkage in the hippocampus, a critical region of the brain that regulates learning and memory. Cortisol also promotes storage of lipids in your fat cells.

Below is a list of physical stressors that can cause your body to hold on to fat.

→ **A very low-calorie diet:** Under 1,200 calories a day for men and 1,000 calories a day for women

→ **Too little dietary fat:** Less than 30 grams a day for men and 20 grams a day for women

→ **Too much negative-accentuated training or other types of exercise:** Longer than 45 minutes per workout or more frequently than two times per week

→ **Too little sleep:** Less than 6 hours per night

→ **Dehydration:** A loss of 1 percent of the body's water can cause alarm.

→ **Excessive heat:** High levels of environmental heat can reduce the body's efficiency.

→ **Accumulated problems:** Business and relationship conflicts can have negative effects.

→ **Sickness, drugs, or extreme behaviors:** Almost anything out of the ordinary can send alarm signals to the body.

As I've pointed out in other chapters, if you want to achieve maximum fat loss, you want to communicate to your body that everything is well. You do this best by avoiding excessive stress and by practicing moderation in almost everything—except the intensity of your negative-accentuated training.

Moderately intense negative training is not very productive. Negative-accentuated training that is performed slowly in the 30-30-30 style is stressful—as it must be—to achieve the fastest possible muscular-growth stimulation. That's why it's important to keep your training brief.

But wait a minute. How does muscular-growth stimulation send a positive message to your system to part with its fat? Once again, we must look to our ancient ancestors for the answer.

Strength and Survival

One of the basic necessities of our ancestors' lives was locomotion, or movement. Movement depended on muscular strength. Anthropological research shows that survival resources were allocated to the muscles first. An individual had to be able to run fast and fight fiercely to eat and avoid being eaten—or to mate or avoid mating, as the case may be. Hard, brief activity produced stronger muscles, and stronger muscles led to success at hunting and in battle, including the battle of the sexes.

Stronger, larger muscles improved the probability of survival.

Today when you go on a moderately reduced-calorie diet, your body perceives stress—that something is wrong. Cortisol is released, which, if sustained long enough, will prevent you from losing fat in the most efficient manner.

To combat this situation, learn to deal with your stressors quickly and productively. Do not let your troubles linger. Be proactive.

And most important, practice overriding your long-term survival mechanisms by stimulating your muscles to grow with negative-accentuated training. But your growing muscles must have a well-rested recovery ability. And well-rested recovery ability is dependent on plenty of sleep.

Then, and only then, will your stimulated muscles draw calories for growth from your fat cells. Doing so significantly increases the effectiveness and efficiency of your ability to reduce fat.

With sleep—especially when it follows negative-accentuated training—more is better, significantly better.

Why don't you sleep on it?

FAT BOMB #7

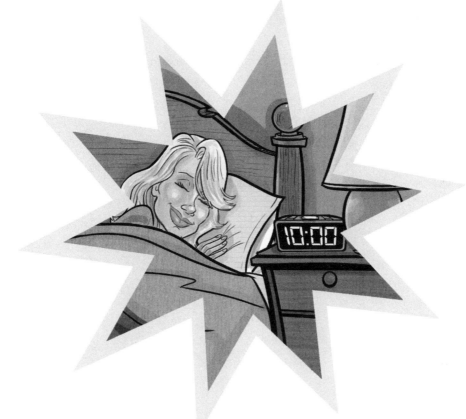

EXTRA SLEEP AND REST

Go to bed an hour earlier each night, but get up at the
same time as always each morning.

DR. PAULA GOLOMBEK
BEFORE & AFTER

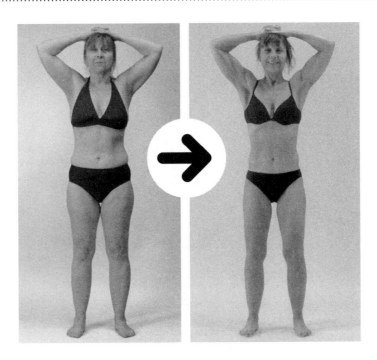

AGE 51, HEIGHT 5'4"

BEFORE BODY WEIGHT

148.2
POUNDS

AFTER BODY WEIGHT

124
POUNDS

AFTER 18 WEEKS

31.93
POUNDS OF FAT LOSS

6.75
INCHES OFF WAIST

7.73
POUNDS OF MUSCLE GAIN

1
INCH ADDED ON UPPER ARMS

FAT BOMB #8:
Social Network Connection

Little tips for losing weight that really add up, plus the benefit of group support

STUDIES show that people who have a strong social network to provide emotional support for their weight-loss effort will lose more pounds than those who try to go it alone. We saw how effective camaraderie and social media could be with our test panels in Gainesville.

Once the Body Fat Breakthrough program began in February 2012, all 65 participants joined a Facebook community specific to our negative-accentuated group. As a group member you could ask questions, report problems, change your workout time, find new recipes, and generally follow the other participants, day by day, as they progressed through the 6-week plan. Socially interacting within this community definitely helped many of the participants maximize their fat-loss and muscle-gain results.

Perhaps there's a fitness center near you that provides similar resources. If not, there are smartphone apps that measure calories consumed, calories burned, and steps taken in walking; record sleep habits; and promote discussions of various fitness topics. If interested, check the following Web sites:

BodyMedia.com

Fitbit.com

GoWearFit.com

HealthTap.com

iHealthLabs.com

Jefit.com

LoseIt.com

LumoBack.com

MyFitnessPal.com

TactioSoft.com

WeightWatchers.com

MensHealth.com

WomensHealthMag.com

My.MensHealth.com/bellyoff

GET CONNECTED

HERE ARE SOME CONCEPTS for getting connected and staying in touch.

- **ORGANIZE A FACEBOOK SITE FOR YOUR FAT-LOSS GROUP.** Use it to schedule training sessions, share new recipes, and post inspirational messages and photos.
- **USE TWITTER TO SHARE DAY-BY-DAY HAPPENINGS.** Tweeting about workouts creates transparency and fosters accountability.
- **CREATE AN ONLINE CALENDAR AND SCHEDULE WORKOUTS AND OTHER ACTIVITIES.** You're not likely to miss a negative workout, a walking session, or a trip to the supermarket if you know others will be expecting you.
- **POST OFTEN ON A MESSAGE BOARD.** Experience back-and-forth discussions, ask questions, share information, and receive support from like-minded people who are involved in a meaningful Web site.

More Lifestyle Tips

A fat bomb doesn't have to be mega-ton huge. Often it's the little things you do that make a big difference in your effort to get back in shape and stick with the lifestyle changes you've adopted. Here are 11 to try out.

1. REBUILD YOUR FOOD ENVIRONMENT

At home, in the office, in your car, rebuild space to help you avoid temptation. Make the easiest choices healthy choices. For example, keep raw vegetables up front and easy to see in the refrigerator. Move the ice cream to the deep freeze in the basement or garage. Customize any personal space to remove tempting items that are off your menu list. Don't buy cookies, candy, and soft drinks. If it's not in your home, you can't eat it.

2. REDUCE YOUR SALT INTAKE

The Food and Nutrition Board's National Research Council recommends 1,100 to 3,300 milligrams of sodium daily for adults. These levels are equivalent to $\frac{1}{2}$ to $1\frac{1}{2}$ teaspoons of table salt. With all the salt used in processed foods, cooking, and salting before eating, most adults consume four to five times this amount.

Aside from the relationship between excessive sodium and high blood pressure, and excessive sodium and fluid retention, salt generally hangs out with high-calorie foods. There seems to be an almost irresistible urge to eat foods that contain salt, fat, and sugar. And once you start, it's difficult to stop.

You can do your part by hiding your saltshaker. I'll do my part by providing you with an eating plan—which includes menus and recipes—that is low in salt.

3. FILL UP ON FIBER

Although fiber is not a nutrient, it can be helpful in fat loss. Fiber, which is the tough, stringy part of plant cells, doesn't nourish your body, because it isn't broken down during digestion. That's the key to its usefulness. Think of fiber as a broom. Its bulk helps sweep the intestines, aiding both digestion and elimination.

The recommended daily fiber intake for adults is 21 to 38 grams, with men needing the higher number. Most adults don't meet those numbers. You'll get more fiber by emphasizing whole wheat breads, whole grain cereals, vegetables, fruits, and legumes.

4. PRACTICE GOOD POSTURE

The act of standing tall burns more calories than does slouching. And standing tall even makes you look leaner. The best posture resembles a marionette with a string attached to the top of its head. Imagine being tugged gently upward by the string. In other words, try to keep the top of your head toward the ceiling. This applies as well to sitting, standing, and walking.

5. BRUSH YOUR TEETH OFTEN

The next time you get the munchies, just try brushing your teeth. It's harder to eat with a clean, minty taste in your mouth. This is especially true if you crave something sweet and you brush with a tingly toothpaste. The taste will temporarily cause anything sweet to taste bitter.

Indeed, you will be enjoying the minty flavor, and any snack would curb this pleasurable sensation. Be sure to rinse well and have some sips of cold water, as well. These serve to further enhance the freshness.

Of course, this is also a reminder to keep a toothbrush handy wherever you happen to be when cravings strike.

6. USE COLOR WISELY

Intense colors can stimulate your appetite. Think about the decorations of your favorite restaurants. They have been carefully selected to promote and enhance your dining experience. Now you want to minimize the effect of color to focus on eating less and losing more fat. Avoid place settings or tablecloths of warm red, orange, bright yellow, or lime green. Even worse may be the red-and-white checkered tablecloths you often see in pizza parlors. You'll eat less on white or pastel plates and tablecloths.

7. CUT BACK ON EVENING TV

Watching television can hypnotize you to the point where you snack and don't realize how much you've eaten. In fact, studies show that people consume

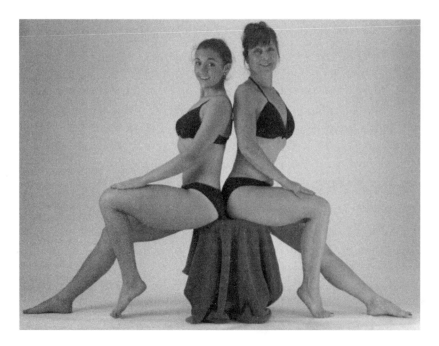

Anya Bernhard, age 17, and her mom, Dr. Paula Golombek, age 51 (see page 210), both did well on the Breakthrough program. As a team, they lost 46 pounds of fat and built 13 pounds of muscle. Their final skin-fold measurements revealed that mother and daughter each had achieved an almost ideal body fat of 15.5 percent.

more calories from snack foods when they watch television. Make it a personal rule never to eat mindlessly while watching TV. Getting outside for a walk, and going to bed an hour earlier will help you break the evening TV habit.

8. BEGIN A HOUSEHOLD PROJECT

To take your mind off food and keep your fingers busy, start a major project around the house. How about painting the guest bedroom, refinishing a table, or even washing and waxing the cars? You will be feeling so smug about finally completing your projects, you will not be upset about missing your usual snack time.

9. TEAM UP WITH A FRIEND

You'll likely get better fat-loss and muscle-gain results if you follow the Body Fat Breakthrough program with a friend. Research shows that accountability keeps people on track. If you work out with a partner, you are less likely to blow off an exercise session.

Both you and your friend should be serious about making a 6-week commitment. The commitment means you'll be exercising together, counting 30-30-30 phases, talking on the phone or texting often, shopping together, walking with each other, and sharing problems.

10. RECOVER QUICKLY

If you blow your eating plan one meal, get back on track the next. Don't say, "Well, I've already blown it—I might as well return to my old ways."

Everyone loses a battle occasionally. Your job is to win the war. And you do that one meal, one day, and one week at a time.

11. BE ASSERTIVE

A leaner and stronger body automatically makes you more assertive. Practice saying no when people offer you certain foods. Practice saying yes to things that are beneficial to your health. Soon you'll be in complete control of your life.

PRACTICE SAYING NO 50 TIMES

NO. NO. NO. NO. NO. NO. No. No. No. No. No. No. No. No. No. No. No. No. No. No. No. No. No. No. Keep on saying no to calorically dense food, to sugary beverages, to your kids' pleadings for candy, to your friend's offer of a slice of death-by-chocolate cake. The more you practice saying no, the easier it will be to say no and the greater self-control you will develop.

This guideline is adapted from a chapter title of the best-selling book *Swim with the Sharks without Being Eaten Alive* by Harvey Mackay.

Says Mackay: "No one ever went broke because he said no too often."

Says Darden: "No one ever lost a significant amount of fat without saying no. Saying no too often will get your fat off even faster."

No. No. No. No. No. No. No. No. No. No. No. No. No. No. No. No. No. No.

FAT BOMB #8

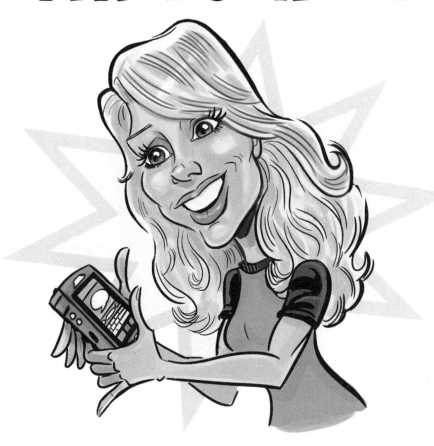

SOCIAL NETWORK CONNECTION

Join a support group that is serious about fat loss and communicate with them on the Internet. Also, check out the latest apps related to fat loss.

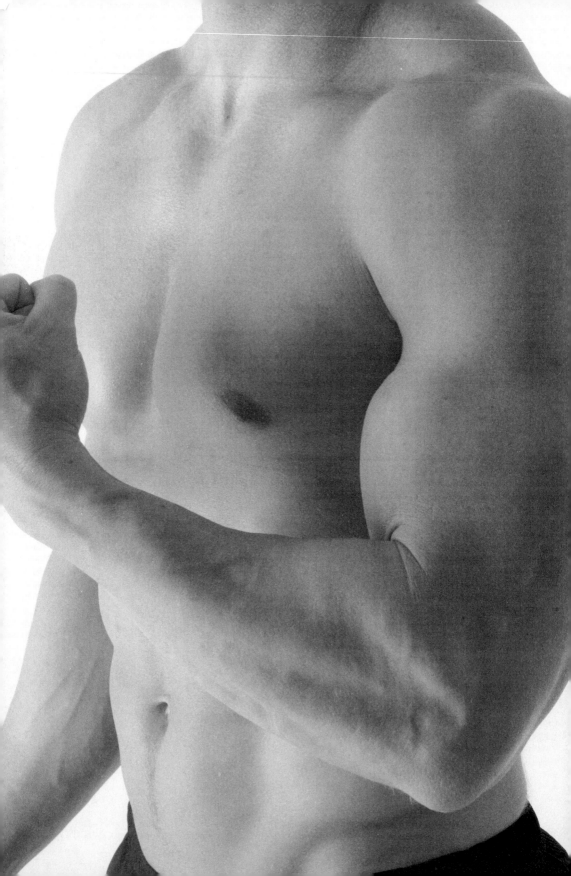

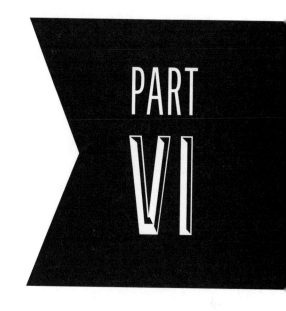

PART
VI

The Breakthrough Program for Fat Loss and Muscle Gain

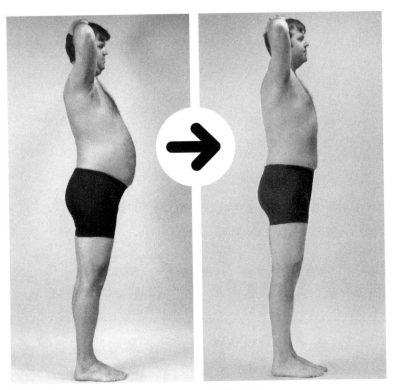

BODY FAT BREAKTHROUGH

JON THOMAS
BEFORE & AFTER

AGE 39, HEIGHT 6'2"

BEFORE BODY WEIGHT

237
POUNDS

AFTER BODY WEIGHT

210.5
POUNDS

AFTER 6 WEEKS

32.5
POUNDS OF FAT LOSS

6
INCHES OFF WAIST

6
POUNDS OF MUSCLE GAIN

GETTING STARTED:
Find Your Baseline

Before you begin,
assess your current condition

YOU probably already know that you have some pounds and inches to lose and some muscle to gain. But you probably don't how to put a number—a realistic number—on what you want to occur throughout your body.

We discussed in Chapter 1 that there's a difference between losing weight and losing fat. And most people specifically need to lose more fat than weight. But determining just how much requires that you put a number on your own fatness. In this chapter, I'll show you how to accurately estimate your fatness with a simple test.

In 6 weeks, will your new body weight accurately reflect the new you? Only in a very general way. It is best to take full-body photographs of yourself, before and after, and compare them with your weight and circumference measurements. I'll show you what I mean by this later.

Do not skip the application of this chapter. Take measurements and photographs before you begin the Breakthrough plan. You'll be glad you did when the pounds and inches start melting away. The Introduction demonstrated that, quite literally, your own mother may not recognize you.

It is most important to have valid measurements. You must follow the recommended guidelines carefully. Be precise and be consistent.

One note: It's difficult to take your own measurements accurately. You'll get truer numbers if you have a dependable partner or friend help you.

Check with Your Physician

Should you call your doctor and schedule a routine physical examination? Actually, because of the prevalence and hazards of obesity in this country, most Americans should get their doctor's permission to *not* exercise and to *not* diet. There is certainly more risk involved in pursuing a sedentary, high-calorie lifestyle. Nevertheless, I recommend that you check with your physician and take this book along with you for easy referral.

A few specific groups of people should not try a reduced-calorie eating plan: children and teenagers; pregnant women; women who are breast-feeding; men and women with certain types of heart, liver, or kidney disease; people with diabetes; and those suffering from some types of arthritis and cancer. Some people should follow a certain program only with their physician's specific guidance. Consult your health-care professional beforehand and play it safe.

Record Your Height and Weight

Remove clothing and shoes and record your height to the nearest quarter inch and your weight to the nearest quarter pound. Be sure to use the same scale when weighing yourself at the end of the plan. For the most accurate recordings, weigh yourself nude in the morning.

Apply Circumference Measurements

These measurements are meaningful because they let you know what is happening in specific areas of your body. Use a plastic tape to measure the following and record your numbers in the blank chart on page 224:

→ Upper arms—hanging and relaxed, midway between the shoulder and elbow

→ Chest—at nipple level

→ 2 inches above navel—belly relaxed

→ At navel level—belly relaxed

→ 2 inches below navel—belly relaxed

→ Hips—at maximum protrusion of buttocks, with feet together

→ Thighs—high, just below the buttocks crease, with legs apart and weight distributed equally on both feet

Do the Pinch Test

You can get a fair estimate of your percentage of body fat by doing the pinch test. For both men and women, this requires taking two measurements, the first one on the back of the upper arm and the second beside the navel. Record the numbers in the blank chart on page 226. Here's the procedure to follow:

→ Locate the first skin-fold site on the back of the right upper arm (triceps area) midway between the shoulder and elbow. Let the arm hang loosely at the side.

→ Grasp a vertical fold of skin between the thumb and first finger. Pull the skin and fat away from the arm. Make sure the fold includes just skin and fat and no muscle.

→ Measure with a ruler the thickness of the skin to the nearest quarter of an inch. Be sure to measure the distance between the thumb and the finger. Sometimes the outer portion of the fold is thicker than the flesh grasped between the fingers. To avoid this, make sure the fold is level with the side of the thumb. Do not press the ruler against

BODY-PART MEASUREMENTS

	BEFORE	AFTER	DIFFERENCE
BODY WEIGHT			
RIGHT UPPER ARM (hanging in middle)			
LEFT UPPER ARM (hanging in middle)			
CHEST (at nipple level)			
2 INCHES ABOVE NAVEL			
AT NAVEL LEVEL			
2 INCHES BELOW NAVEL			
HIPS (at largest protrusion)			
RIGHT THIGH (just below buttocks crease)			
LEFT THIGH (just below buttocks crease)			

the skin. This will flatten the skin and make it appear thicker than it really is.

→ Take two separate measurements of the triceps skin-fold thickness, releasing the skin between each measure, and record the average of the two.

→ Locate the second skin-fold site, which is immediately adjacent to the right side of the navel.

→ Grasp a vertical fold of skin between the thumb and first finger and follow the same technique as previously described.

→ Take two separate measurements of the abdominal skin-fold thickness and record the average of the two.

→ Add the average triceps skin-fold measurement to the average abdominal skin-fold measurement. This is your combined total.

→ Estimate the percentage of body fat from the chart on page 226 and record it with the pinch-test measurements.

→ Determine fat loss at the end of 6 weeks by multiplying the percentage of body fat times body weight for the before-and-after tests. For example, if a woman weighs 168 pounds with 28 percent body fat at the start of the program, that's 47.04 pounds of fat. If she completes the program at 150 pounds with 18 percent body fat, that's 27 pounds of fat. The difference between 47.04 and 27 is 20.04 pounds.

→ Calculate the amount of muscle gain by subtracting the weight loss from the fat loss. In the example above, where fat loss equals 20.04 pounds and weight loss is 18 pounds, 2.04 pounds of muscle are gained.

Fat composes more than 25 percent of the body weight of most Americans. An ideal amount of body fat for most men is 12 percent. The average woman's ideal status is 18 percent. Lean, athletic men and women may desire to lower their ideal figures by another 5 or 6 percentage points.

PINCH-TEST MEASUREMENTS

	BEFORE	AFTER
RIGHT TRICEPS		
RIGHT ABDOMINAL		
TOTAL		
BODY-FAT PERCENTAGE		
FAT POUNDS		

ESTIMATED PERCENTAGE OF BODY FAT

SKIN-FOLD THICKNESS (TRICEPS PLUS ABDOMINAL)	PERCENT FAT (MEN)	PERCENT FAT (WOMEN)
¾ INCH	5–9	8–13
1 INCH	9–13	13–18
1¼ INCHES	13–18	18–23
1½ INCHES	18–22	23–28
1¾ INCHES	22–27	28–33
2¼ INCHES	27–32	33–38
2¾ INCHES	32–37	38–43

Take Full-Body Photographs

There is no better way to evaluate your current condition than to have full-body photographs taken of yourself in a small, revealing bathing suit. Here are the best procedures to follow:

- → Wear a solid-color bathing suit or bikini.

- → Stand against an uncluttered, light-colored background.

- → Have the person with the camera move away from you until he or she can see your entire body in the viewfinder. It's best to be 15 to 20 feet from the subject and zoom in with the camera lens. The camera should be turned sideways for a vertical format. It's also best for the photographer to be seated with the camera approximately 3 feet off the floor.

- → Stand relaxed for three pictures: front, right side, and back. Do not try to suck in your stomach.

- → Interlace your fingers and place them on top of your head, so the contours of your torso will be plainly visible. Keep your feet 8 inches apart for the front and back shots but together on the side picture.

- → Download the digital before photos into your computer. Crop the best ones tightly to 4 inches by 6 inches size.

- → Retake the photos 6 weeks later, following the same directions, with the same bathing suit and camera.

- → Download your after images into your computer.

- → Crop and make the prints the same size as the before ones. Your height in both sets of photos should be precisely the same, so more valid comparisons can be made.

Set Realistic Goals

Taking your before measurements and full-body photographs will help you determine realistic goals for your Body Fat Breakthrough plan. The success stories throughout this book will also help.

The following averages provide specific pounds and inches lost. They were compiled from before-and-after measurements of 118 people (41 men and 77 women) who went through one or more phases of the Body Fat Breakthrough course at Gainesville Health & Fitness in 2012.

Each man lost, in 6 weeks, an average of:
  27.5 pounds of fat
  5.1 inches off the waist
Each woman lost, in 6 weeks, an average of:
  15.5 pounds of fat
  4 inches off the waist

The same men added an average of *8 pounds of muscle* to their physiques. The women gained an average of *4.6 pounds of muscle* per woman.

These numbers provide realistic goals for most men and women motivated to follow the Breakthrough plan for 6 weeks. Some individuals will achieve lower results, while some can achieve greater results—as much as 75 percent above the averages.

Be Prepared

One of my favorite quotes from a wise old-school coach, Benjamin Franklin, seems appropriate here:

If you fail to prepare, prepare to fail.

Here are a few more important steps to take in preparation, plus a brief summary of key Fat Bombs that make up the Body Fat Breakthrough program:

Purchase measuring spoons and cups and a small scale. Most people tend to overestimate 1 ounce of cheese, 2 ounces of chicken breast, or 4 ounces of orange juice. Such practices lead to inaccurate calorie counting and ineffective fat loss. It's important to become familiar with and correctly use measuring spoons, cups, and food scales.

All the items can be purchased inexpensively at your local supermarket or department store. With the food scale, however, you'd be wise to spend more money and buy a battery-operated digital scale instead of the less-expensive spring-loaded type.

Take a vitamin/mineral tablet each day. During the program, I recommend that you take one multiple vitamin with minerals each morning with breakfast. Make sure that no nutrient listed on the label exceeds 100 percent of the Recommended Dietary Allowance. High-potency supplements are not necessary.

Examine the menus, recipes, and shopping lists. Glance through the menus, recipes, and shopping lists beginning on page 236 for an overview of what you'll be eating during the next 6 weeks. Your results will be more effective if you plan ahead.

Follow the carbohydrate-rich, descending-calorie eating plan. Remember, carbohydrates are your body's primary source of energy, as well as an important vehicle for the intake of many vitamins and minerals. Approximately 50 percent of your daily calories are from carbohydrate-rich foods on the Breakthrough plan. The remaining 50 percent of the calories are equally divided between proteins and fats. The 50-25-25 ratio of carbohydrates, proteins, and fats is ideal for maximum fat loss and muscle gain. Furthermore, such a breakdown—with slight modifications—can be continued for a lifetime of healthy eating.

Many overfat men and women make the mistake of immediately reducing their dietary calories from a typical 3,000 to 1,200 or fewer a day. Such a drastic cut in calories can cause at least three problems. First, after several days you may get an uncontrollable appetite, which causes you to break the diet. Second, a drastic reduction in calories may actually cause your body to preserve its fat stores. Third, your body starts conserving energy and burns fewer and fewer calories. As a result, you'll have to reduce your calories even more to keep losing. Such extremely low-calorie diets are doomed to self-destruct.

I've found through my research that you can prevent all of these problems by reducing your calories in a gradual manner. That's exactly what the Body Fat Breakthrough program does.

During weeks 1 and 2, men start with 1,600 calories per day, and women begin with 1,400 calories per day. For weeks 3 and 4, the calories drop to 1,500 per day for men and 1,300 per day for women. For weeks 5 and 6, there's another reduction of 100 calories: 1,400 per day for men and 1,200 per day for women.

At 1,600 calories a day for a man and 1,400 calories a day for a woman, you won't develop a ravenous appetite, nor will your body be stressed into its preservation stages. Quite the opposite will happen. Your body will become more efficient at burning fat.

Eat smaller meals more frequently. You'll consume six small meals each day, with approximately $2\frac{1}{2}$ hours between each meal. The only difference

VEGETABLES: CANNED, FROZEN, OR FRESH?

THERE IS A COMMON BELIEF THAT fresh vegetables are nutritionally superior to canned or frozen vegetables. While this belief may have been based on fact years ago, the sophisticated methods of food preservation applied in the last decade lead to different conclusions.

In today's canning process, the vegetable is harvested at the proper time to assure optimal size, appearance, and nutritional value. The product is chilled immediately after picking and rushed to the factory. Once at the factory, it is washed and blanched and immediately processed by a short-term, high-temperature method. This cooking technique, followed by a rapid cooling period, is the key to the superiority of industrial procedures over most home methods.

If the can is opened at home, it is necessary only to warm the food prior to serving. Furthermore, manufacturers now offer a wide variety of canned vegetables with *no salt added, no sugar added,* and *no preservatives added.* In the freezing process, if vegetables are picked and then quick-frozen, the nutritional values are equal to or slightly higher than those of fresh vegetables.

Freshly harvested vegetables cooked immediately do not have significantly greater nutritional value than canned or frozen vegetables. Slow-cooking methods used at home often destroy more vitamins than are lost during the industrial processing. In fact, vegetables that are poorly stored at the market may be less nutritious than those picked from a home garden. Vegetables that are locally grown in season are frequently cheaper than commercially processed vegetables. But sometimes, even when they're in season, fresh vegetables can be more expensive than canned or frozen ones.

From a nutritional viewpoint, it really doesn't matter whether you consume canned, frozen, or fresh vegetables. They are all rich in nutrients.

between the eating plan for men and women is that men add 100 calories to each lunch and 100 calories to each dinner selection.

The menus and recipes in the next chapter have all been simplified. All you have to do is read and follow the easy-to-understand directions.

Drink 128 ounces of cold water each day. Do not underestimate the importance of drinking 1 gallon of cold water each day. Invariably, the individuals who lose the most fat in 6 weeks are the most consistent with their water drinking.

A 32-ounce insulated plastic bottle with a straw makes this step easier to follow. Most people find they can consume more fluid with a straw than they can by drinking from a glass. A great way to keep up with your superhydration is to place rubber bands around the middle of the bottle equal to the number of bottles you are supposed to drink. Each time you finish 32 ounces, take off a rubber band.

Apply negative-accentuated training twice or once a week. The Body Fat Breakthrough Program applies negative-accentuated training twice a week for the first 3 weeks and once a week for the last 3 weeks. As your calories descend with each 2 weeks, the number of negative-accentuated exercises in your workouts gradually ascends.

Use the cold plunge after your workout. If you have access to a cold plunge after your negative-accentuated training, by all means use it for 5 to 10 minutes. If not, consider trying a U-shaped ice pack around your neck, as I describe in Chapter 5; even a cold shower might be an alternative, which I also discuss in the same chapter.

Walk after your evening meal. You'll burn more calories if you take a leisurely walk after your evening meal each day. Remember, you should begin the walk within 15 minutes after the meal and continue for only 30 minutes.

Sleep an extra hour each night. Getting extra sleep will absolutely help your fat-loss and muscle-gain results. The recommended way is to retire an hour earlier each night but arise at the usual time each morning.

Avoid overstress. Generally speaking, you want to stay clear of extremes. Send as many messages as you can to your body that everything is okay, standard, and tranquil. Do not get stressed out. Stay calm. Under such conditions, you will freely pull calories from your fat cells.

You are now well prepared to begin the Body Fat Breakthrough program.

The next 6 weeks will make a difference in your life. Be patient.

Don't be surprised if, 6 weeks from today, everybody around you is talking about your great-looking body!

THERESA FORTE
BEFORE & AFTER

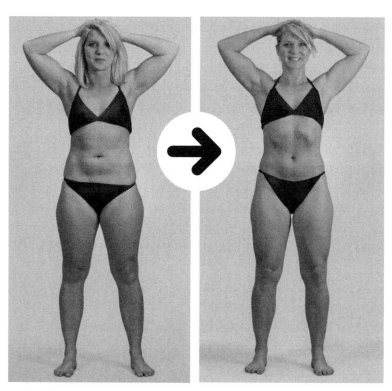

AGE 27, HEIGHT 5'3"

BEFORE BODY WEIGHT

155
POUNDS

AFTER BODY WEIGHT

145
POUNDS

AFTER 6 WEEKS

18.74
POUNDS OF FAT LOSS

3.625
INCHES OFF WAIST

8.74
POUNDS OF MUSCLE GAIN

CHAPTER
25

Your Diet Plan for Weeks 1 to 6

Prepare to eat smaller meals more often

THE food that you choose to swallow has a huge impact on your weight and fitness level. Just how much you consume has an even greater influence on your body shape, which is why calorie restriction is a big part of this book's program. The nutrition advice and specific menus in the Body Fat Breakthrough eating plan are designed for maximum fat loss. For best results, follow them exactly. You will need to cut calories to achieve the results you want, but that doesn't mean you'll starve. In fact, my plan will keep your hunger satisfied in such a way that you will never feel as if you are sacrificing a good meal.

I've made every attempt to use current, popular brand names and calorie counts, which are listed in the menus. But as you probably know, products are often changed and discontinued. If a listed product is not available in your area for whatever reason, you'll have to substitute with something similar. Become a label reader at your supermarket.

Each day you will choose from a limited selection of foods for breakfast and lunch. One of the easiest ways to stick to a smart nutrition program is to reduce your choices and opportunities for temptation. Simplify your diet and you'll make it that much easier on yourself. I've found that most adults can consume the same basic breakfast and lunch for months with little, or no, modification. By adding ample variety during your evening meal, you can easily overcome same-food boredom and make daily eating interesting and enjoyable. Additionally, the eating plan includes a midmorning, midafternoon, and late-night snack to keep your energy high and eliminate hunger pangs.

Begin week 1 on Monday and continue through Sunday. Week 2 is a repeat of week 1. Calories for each food are noted in parentheses. A shopping list follows at the end of the chapter.

Guidelines for the Menus

→ Each daily menu consists of six small meals of 100 to 400 calories each. During weeks 1 and 2, women consume 1,400 calories per day and men eat 1,600 calories a day.

Note: *During weeks 3 and 4, the calories drop to 1,300 per day for women and 1,500 per day for men. For weeks 5 and 6, there's another reduction of 100 calories: 1,200 per day for women and 1,400 per day for men.*

→ The only difference between the eating plan for women and men is that men add 100 calories each to their lunch and dinner.

→ Noncaloric beverages are any type of water—tap, bottled, carbonated, or flavored—with no calories, as well as zero-calorie soft drinks. It's okay to have 1 or 2 cups of regular coffee or tea per day.

→ For the latest frozen, microwaveable meals and for possible dinner substitutions, please refer to the following Web sites: Michelinas.com; HealthyChoice.com; and LeanCuisine.com.

→ For meal-replacement shake mixes, try:
   • *Metabolic Drive (Award Winning) Formula (MetabolicDrive.com; under Store, click Supplements)*
   • *Myoplex Original (EAS.com)*
   • *Making your own using whey protein powder—find recipes at MensHealth.com and WomensHealthMag.com*

MEN: CONSUMING SIX MEALS A DAY FOR 1,600 CALORIES

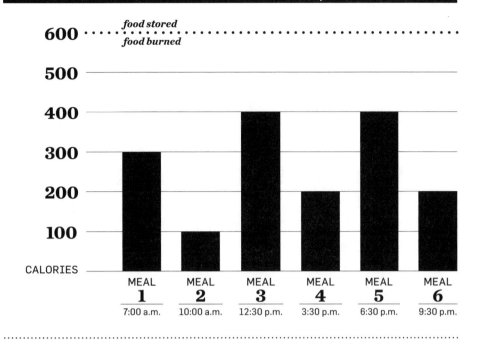

WOMEN: CONSUMING SIX MEALS A DAY FOR 1,400 CALORIES

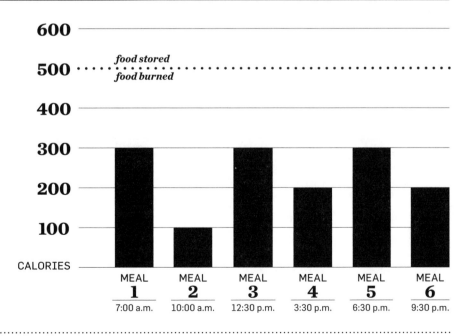

Menus

WEEKS 1 AND 2

Women consume 1,400 calories a day.

Men consume 1,600 calories a day.

BREAKFAST = 300 CALORIES

Choose one—bagel, cereal, or shake—and a noncaloric beverage.

1	Thomas' Hearty Grains whole wheat bagel (240)
1	ounce light cream cheese (60)

or

1	cup Kashi GOLEAN cereal (140)
½	cup fat-free milk (45) or 1 cup almond milk (40)
1	large banana (8¾" long) (100)

or

2	scoops Metabolic Drive Formula shake mix (220) or other meal replacement to equal the appropriate calories
1	large banana (8¾" long) (100)
12	ounces cold water

Place in blender and mix until smooth.

MIDMORNING SNACK = 100 CALORIES

Choose one of the following:

1	cup light, fat-free, flavored yogurt (100)
14	whole, unsalted almonds (100)
1	apple (3" diameter) (100)
2	cups light microwave popcorn (100)

LUNCH = 300 CALORIES

Choose one—sandwich or soup—and a noncaloric beverage.

Ham or turkey sandwich (300 calories) made with:

2	slices whole wheat bread (140)
1–2	tablespoons classic mustard (0)
3	ounces deli-type ham or turkey, sliced thin (90)
1	ounce fat-free cheese (1½ slices) (50)
2	slices tomato (10)
2	lettuce leaves (10)

or

Healthy Choice Soup, Chicken & Dumplings—entire can (300)

MEN ADD 100 CALORIES:

8	ounces V8 100% vegetable juice (50)
7	whole unsalted almonds (50)

MIDAFTERNOON SNACK = 200 CALORIES

Choose two:

1	cup light, fat-free, flavored yogurt (100)
1	Breakstone's 100-Calorie Cottage Doubles, various flavors (100)
14	whole, unsalted almonds (100)
1	apple (3" diameter) (100)
2	cups light microwave popcorn (100)

DINNER = 300 CALORIES

I've successfully used the frozen dinners listed below—or earlier versions of them—in my weight-loss programs for more than 20 years. I like them because they make portion control easy by delivering the ideal portion of selected foods. Consuming these microwaveable frozen dinners during weeks 1 and 2 of the program makes portion control a no-brainer, and you start to learn what 300 calories looks like—without doing the weighing and measuring, which is a big turnoff for a lot of people. So I recommend you try the frozen dinners during the first 2 weeks of the plan. Fresh, whole foods are always better than processed foods—no doubt about that—but when it comes to learning new lifestyle habits involving your diet, tricks like this can be very helpful. Don't worry—during weeks 3 and 4, we introduce some fresh food substitutions, which will involve some weighing and measuring. But for now, make it easy on yourself. You have enough to think about without having to worry about measuring proper calorie portions.

Choose one of these frozen, microwaveable meals and a noncaloric beverage.

Orange Chicken, Lean Cuisine Culinary Collection (300)

Lemon Pepper Fish, Lean Cuisine Culinary Collection (290)

Steak Tips Dijon, Lean Cuisine Dinnertime Cuisine (280)

Three Cheese Ziti, Michelina's Lean Gourmet (290)

MEN ADD 100 CALORIES:

$1\frac{1}{2}$ slices whole wheat bread (105)

EVENING SNACK = 200 CALORIES
Choose two:

1   cup light, fat-free, flavored yogurt (100)

1   Breakstone's 100-Calorie Cottage Doubles, various flavors (100)

14   whole, unsalted almonds (100)

1   apple (3" diameter) (100)

2   cups light microwave popcorn (100)

SUBSTITUTIONS FOR WEEKS 3 AND 4 AND FOR WEEKS 5 AND 6

Women:

Weeks 3 and 4 = 1,300 calories a day: Eliminate one midafternoon snack (–100 calories) from weeks 1 and 2 menus.

Weeks 5 and 6 = 1,200 calories a day: Eliminate one evening snack (–100 calories) from weeks 3 and 4 menus.

Men:

Weeks 3 and 4 = 1,500 calories a day: Eliminate one midafternoon snack (–100 calories) from weeks 1 and 2 menus.

Weeks 5 and 6 = 1,400 calories a day: Eliminate one evening snack (–100 calories) from weeks 3 and 4 menus.

SUBSTITUTIONS FOR A 300-CALORIE LUNCH DURING WEEKS 3 THROUGH 6

Chef's Salad (306)

In a large bowl, mix the following:

- 2 cups chopped lettuce (20)
- 2 ounces white meat, chicken or turkey (80)
- 2 ounces fat-free cheese (100)
- 4 slices tomato, chopped (28)
- 1 tablespoon fat-free dressing (8)
- 1 slice whole wheat bread, toasted (70)

Sandwich from Subway (300)

6" Turkey Breast & Black Forest Ham on 9-grain wheat bread with plenty of raw vegetables and no oil-based dressings

SUBSTITUTIONS FOR A 100-CALORIE SNACK

Fruits

- 5 dried prunes (100)
- 1 ounce raisins (82)
- 1/2 cantaloupe (5" diameter) (94)

Energy Bars

Most of the popular energy bars—such as Zone, PowerBar, Odwalla, and Clif—may be used as snacks. Their calories, however, range from 210 to 240, so slightly less than one-half bar may be applied as one selection.

Tuna Salad (260)

In a large bowl, mix the following:

- ½ can (2.5 ounces) chunk light tuna in water (50)
- ½ cup (4 ounces) whole kernel corn, canned, no salt added (60)
- ½ cup (4 ounces) canned sweet peas (60)
- 2 tablespoons sweet pickle relish (40)
- 1 tablespoon Hellmann's Light Mayonnaise (50)
- 1 tablespoon Dijon mustard (0)

Mahi Mahi and Broccoli (295)

- 4 ounces mahi mahi fish, grilled (120)
- 1 cup broccoli, sautéed in 1 teaspoon olive oil (70)
- 1½ slices whole wheat bread (105)

Spice-Rubbed Fresh Tuna Tacos with Cilantro-Avocado-Lime Cream (316)

- ¼ teaspoon ground cumin (2)
- ¼ teaspoon chili powder (4)
- ⅛ teaspoon garlic powder (1)
- Salt, to taste (0)
- Black pepper, to taste (0)
- 1 (4-ounce) tuna steak (123)
- ¼ Hass avocado (57)
- 1 tablespoon loosely packed fresh cilantro leaves (0)
- 1 tablespoon light sour cream (18)
- ¾ teaspoon lime juice (1)
- 2 corn tortillas (105)
- ¼ white onion, thinly sliced (5)

Combine the cumin, chili powder, garlic powder, and half of the salt, and pepper in a bowl. Rub over the tuna steaks and let stand for 10 minutes.

Meanwhile, combine the avocado, cilantro, sour cream, lime juice, and remaining salt in a food processor and puree. Preheat a ridged grill pan that has been coated with cooking spray. Add the tuna and cook 2 to 3 minutes per side, or until well marked and cooked through. Transfer to a cutting board. Thinly slice the tuna. Heat tortillas over a gas burner, turning occasionally, about 1 minute, or place the tortillas between clean paper towels and microwave on high for 15 to 20 seconds to warm. Fill the tortillas with sliced tuna and onion and top with the cilantro-avocado cream.

Chicken Fajita (318)

Butter-flavored cooking spray (0)
$1/2$ tablespoon low-calorie margarine (25)
4 ounces (raw weight) boneless, skinless chicken strips (160)
$1/4$ cup onion slices (11)
$1/4$ cup green bell pepper strips (5)
$1/4$ cup red bell pepper strips (6)
1 flour tortilla (6") (94)
1 tablespoon Worcestershire sauce (15)
$1/4$ fresh lemon wedge (2)

Coat a nonstick skillet with cooking spray. Add the margarine and melt. Brown the chicken in the skillet until no longer pink in the center. Remove the chicken and drain on paper towels. Add the onion and peppers and sauté until tender. Return the chicken to the skillet and cook thoroughly. Just before serving, heat the tortilla. Add the Worcestershire sauce to the chicken-vegetable mixture and toss. Squeeze on the juice of the lemon and toss again.

Place the heated tortilla on a dinner plate. Place the chicken-vegetable mixture on one side and fold over. Serve immediately.

Crab-Stuffed Potato (314)

1 medium ($2^1/2$" × $4^3/4$") baking potato (173)
Butter-flavored cooking spray (0)
3 ounces chopped imitation crabmeat (82)
$1/4$ cup low-fat (1%) cottage cheese (40)
1 tablespoon fat-free plain yogurt (8)
2 tablespoons chopped onion (6)
2 tablespoons chopped red bell pepper (3)
$1/4$ lemon wedge (2)
Paprika

Scrub the potato well and allow it to dry. Pierce with a fork several times. Spray a small amount of cooking spray on the potato and distribute it evenly with your hand. Place the potato on a paper towel and microwave on high for 4 to 5 minutes. Let stand for 2 minutes.

Cut the potato in half lengthwise. Scoop the pulp from each half into a small bowl, leaving a $1/2$" thick shell. Set aside the potato halves.

Mash the potato well. Add the crabmeat, cottage cheese, yogurt, onion, bell pepper, and juice of the lemon to the mashed potato. Mix until smooth. Spoon into the shells and sprinkle with paprika.

Place the stuffed potato on a plate, microwave on high for 1 minute, and serve.

300-Calorie Hamburger (309)

   4 ounces extra-lean (95% lean) ground beef (155)
      Butter-flavored cooking spray (0)
   1 whole wheat bun (look for Cobblestone or Pepperidge Farm) (120)
   1 tablespoon mustard (0)
   1 tablespoon sweet pickle relish (20)
   1 slice ($\frac{1}{8}$") raw onion (6)
   2 thin slices tomato (6)
   2 lettuce leaves (2)

Flatten the ground beef into a patty. Coat a nonstick skillet with cooking spray. Cook the patty on medium heat and place on paper towels.

Toast the bun. Spread the top half with the mustard and relish. Place the patty, onion, tomato, and lettuce, on the bottom half, cover with the top half, and serve.

Quick Pork Chops with Green Salsa (239)

   6 tablespoons frozen shelled edamame (75)
   1 boneless pork chop (3 ounces), trimmed of all visible fat (108)
   $\frac{1}{4}$ teaspoon ground cumin (2)
      Salt, to taste (0)
   $\frac{3}{4}$ teaspoon canola oil (31)
   $1\frac{1}{2}$ tomatillos, cut into wedges (16)
   1 scallions, cut into $\frac{1}{2}$" pieces (5)
   $\frac{1}{8}$ teaspoon minced garlic (1)
   2 tablespoons fat-free, reduced-sodium chicken broth (1)
   1 tablespoon chopped cilantro (0)

Prepare the edamame according to package directions; drain.

Meanwhile, rub the chops with the cumin and salt. Coat a large nonstick skillet with cooking spray and heat over medium-high heat. Add the chops and cook for 4 minutes, turning once, or until a thermometer inserted in the center of a chop registers 160°F and the juices run clear. Remove to a plate and keep warm.

Heat the oil in the same skillet over medium-high heat. Cook the tomatillos, scallions, and garlic, stirring constantly, for 5 minutes, or until browned. Add the broth, cilantro, and edamame and cook for 3 minutes, or until the flavors meld. Serve with the chops.

Note: To the above seven fresh-food meals, men add 100 calories. The 100 calories can be the appropriate amounts of any of the following: whole wheat bread, apple slices, grapes, or other fruits.

SHOPPING LIST FOR WEEKS 1 AND 2 MENUS

The quantities for one week of the listed foods will depend on your specific selections. Review your choices and adjust the shopping list accordingly. Remember to check nutrition information on products you buy so that you can carefully follow the serving sizes in the menus. It may be helpful for you to photocopy this list each week before doing your shopping.

STAPLES

Mustard

Meal replacement shakes

Fat-free milk or almond milk

Whole, unsalted almonds

Noncaloric beverages: water, diet soft drinks, tea, and coffee

GRAINS

Thomas' Hearty Grains whole wheat bagels

Kashi GOLEAN cereal

Whole wheat bread

Light microwave popcorn

FRUITS

Apples (3" diameter)

Bananas

VEGETABLES

Lettuce

Tomatoes

V-8 100% vegetable juice

DAIRY

Light cream cheese

Fat-free cheese

Light, fat-free, flavored yogurt

Breakstone's 100-Calorie Cottage Doubles

MEAT AND ENTRÉES

White turkey meat, thin sliced

Ham, thin sliced

Frozen, microwaveable dinners or entrées

- *Orange Chicken, Lean Cuisine Culinary Collection*
- *Lemon Pepper Fish, Lean Cuisine Culinary Collection*
- *Steak Tips Dijon, Lean Cuisine Dinnertime Cuisine*
- *Three Cheese Ziti, Michelina's Lean Gourmet*
- *Chicken & Dumplings, Healthy Choice Soup (can)*

ANYA BERNHARD
BEFORE & AFTER

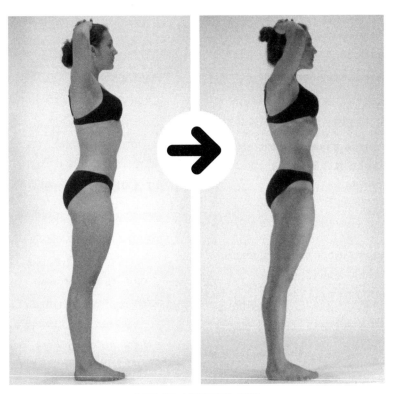

AGE 17, HEIGHT 5'6"

BEFORE BODY WEIGHT

137.8
POUNDS

AFTER BODY WEIGHT

128.8
POUNDS

AFTER 6 WEEKS

14
POUNDS OF FAT LOSS

3.5
INCHES OFF WAIST

5
POUNDS OF MUSCLE GAIN

CHAPTER

26

Your Negative Workout Routines

Apply the positive from the negative and build bigger, stronger muscles to transform your body from flabby to fit

FROM previous chapters, you should be convinced that negative-accentuated training is the best type of muscle-building exercise for fat loss. Larger, stronger muscles trigger fat loss uniquely by requiring more calories during rest and recovery as well as when you're actually doing the sweating. This chapter outlines the three phases of the 6-week program, detailing each of the recommended workouts.

Precision Guidelines

Spend several minutes looking over the exercises listed in the various routines in this chapter. Each exercise is detailed and illustrated in Chapter 16.

Choose between body-weight movements and free-weight/ machine exercises. If you train at home, you may want to apply body-weight movements. If you belong to a commercial fitness center or gym, you'll probably have access to free weights and machines. Most of the women and men involved in my Breakthrough test program used a combination of free-weight and machine exercises.

Select the appropriate resistance. Initially, it's important that you learn how to perform each exercise correctly. You'll learn better if the resistance is not too heavy or too light. Try to select a moderate resistance at first, something you can do easily for 20-20-20: Twenty seconds on the negative, 20 seconds on the positive, and 20 seconds on the negative. Remember, in most negative-accentuated exercises, it's time under load that's most important, not the number of repetitions you do. After the first week, increase the resistance so that 20-20-20 is challenging.

Control your movements. Rushing each exercise diminishes results and can cause injury. Keep a watch with a second hand in plain sight so you can keep your time under load at the called-for number.

Count the seconds of each stroke. Start with 20-20-20 and record the actual number of seconds you make with each negative-positive-negative phase. When you can do 30-30-30, increase the resistance by 5 to 10 percent at the next workout and continue in your progression.

Expect some soreness. Soreness in exercised body parts is an indication that you've stretched and contracted little-used muscles. Expect some soreness after each of your workouts, especially those that involve new exercises.

Decrease your frequency. The idea is to do less as you get stronger. For the first 3 weeks, you'll do the resistance training workout twice weekly, which means training sessions on Monday and Thursday, or on Tuesday and Friday. During weeks 4, 5, and 6, the negative-accentuated training is reduced to only once a week. That's right, you'll continue to get the same benefits but for less time and work! Once-a-week training will be ideal for at least a year, at which time you may choose to go on a routine of once every 10 days.

Body-Weight Routines

The following body-weight routines are designed for use at home. They were also tested on small groups of exercisers at Gainesville Health & Fitness. They work well in both situations.

The routines are divided into three phases: weeks 1 and 2, weeks 3 and 4, and weeks 5 and 6. The eight recommended negative-accentuated body-weight exercises are described and illustrated in Chapter 16.

WEEKS 1 AND 2

Squat	Chinup between Chair Backs
Bottom-Emphasized Calf Raise	L-Seat Dip
Pushup	Situp

WEEKS 3 AND 4

Squat	L-Seat Dip
Bottom-Emphasized Calf Raise	Situp
Pushup	Side Crunch*
Chinup between Chair Backs	

WEEKS 5 AND 6

Squat	L-Seat Dip
Bottom-Emphasized Calf Raise	Situp
Pushup	Side Crunch
Chinup between Chair Backs	Back Raise*

New exercise

Free-Weight/Machine Routines

For these routines, you'll need access to barbells, dumbbells, and some basic exercise machines—such as Nautilus, Cybex, Hammer, or MedX—which are found in fitness centers throughout the United States and Canada. Where there is a choice of exercises, alternate between them or use one or the other.

WEEKS 1 AND 2

Leg Curl

Leg Press (or Barbell Squat)

Chest Press (or Barbell Bench Press)

Lat Machine Pulldown

Dumbbell Triceps Extension

Situp on Declined Board

WEEKS 3 AND 4

Leg Curl

Leg Extension*

Leg Press (or Barbell Squat)

Chest Press (or Barbell Bench Press)

Lat Machine Pulldown

Dumbbell Triceps Extension

Barbell Curl*

Situp on Declined Board

New exercise

WEEKS 5 AND 6

Leg Curl

Leg Extension

Leg Press (or Barbell Squat)

Chest Press (or Barbell Bench Press or Negative-Only Dip*)

Lat Machine Pulldown (or Negative-Only Chinup*)

Barbell Overhead Press*

Barbell Shoulder Shrug*

Dumbbell Triceps Extension

Barbell Curl

Situp on Declined Board

New exercise

Note: All of the above negative-accentuated free-weight and machine exercises are described and illustrated in Chapter 16.

Charting Your Progress

Keep accurate records of all your workouts. The following routine chart has room for 10 exercises, with space to the right to note your resistance and time under load for the workouts that are spread over 6 weeks.

Make two copies of this page. Fill in the blanks at the top. List your exercises in the left column. Now you're ready to progress through the routines.

THE BODY FAT BREAKTHROUGH WORKOUT CARD

EXERCISE	DATE						
	BODY WEIGHT						
1.							
2.							
3.							
4.							
5.							
6.							
7.							
8.							
9.							
10.							

JEREMY LEON
BEFORE & AFTER

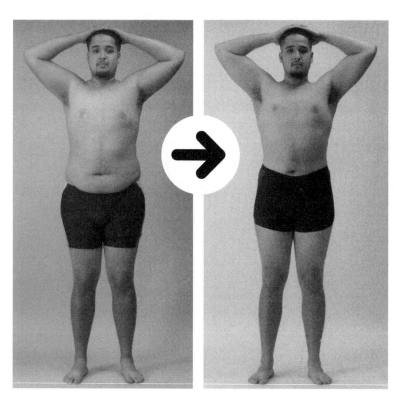

AGE 22, HEIGHT 5'11"

BEFORE BODY WEIGHT

245
POUNDS

AFTER BODY WEIGHT

205
POUNDS

AFTER 18 WEEKS

58.8
POUNDS OF FAT LOSS

9
INCHES OFF WAIST

18.8
POUNDS OF MUSCLE GAIN

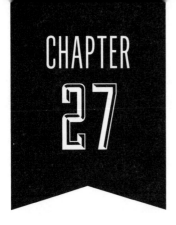
Troubleshooting

A little knowledge can help you overcome challenges

DURING the first month of any new eating and exercising plan, certain situations may arise that cause hesitancy and doubt. For example, among our test panel, several people asked about the popular low-carbohydrate diets. Why weren't low-carbohydrate diets an option? Then there was a common desire to know how to eat when on a vacation or during a holiday party. Others were looking for guidance for eating at restaurants.

The following troubleshooting guide will help you prepare for these and other challenges to your progress.

Low-Carbohydrate Diets

Some of the Gainesville participants followed low-carbohydrate eating plans before they embarked on the Body Fat Breakthrough program, so there was concern. Generally, there are two schools of thought on food and the process of weight loss:

- → **Calories count:** The first school contends that the law of conservation of energy governs weight loss. In other words, to maintain weight, the energy your body uses through heat given off and physical work done must equal the calories you consume as food, because the measure of energy is a calorie. If you take in more energy than your body uses, you gain weight, and vice versa.

- → **Carbohydrates count:** The second school argues that certain foods or food combinations—namely, elimination of carbohydrates and replacement with fats and proteins—have special qualities that cause faster weight loss. Calories aren't a critical factor in this position. More important is to, say, replace carbohydrates with fats and proteins, because they help you avoid weight gain and promote fat loss, or so the theory goes.

Important: Anyone who appreciates science and examines the evidence from both schools of thought soon realizes that human metabolism must obey the law of conservation of energy—as does everything else in nature. Isaac Newton initially recognized conservation of energy in 1687, and numerous other scientists, such as Max Rubner, Wilbur Atwater, Francis Benedict, and Albert Einstein, confirmed the validity of the concept in the early 20th century.

All dietary calories—in the form of carbohydrates, fats, and proteins—do indeed count in the fat-loss game.

THE REAL FACTS

The following 10 bullets briefly review the problems associated with low-carbohydrate dieting:

- → The initial weight loss from a low-carbohydrate diet is mostly water, not fat. Without carbohydrates, the body quickly depletes the sugar (glucose and glycogen) stored in the muscles and liver. Each ounce of sugar carries with it 3 ounces of water. It's not unusual for a dieter to utilize 2 pounds of sugar in the first 4 to 5 days on this kind of diet. Thus, 2 pounds of sugar + 6 pounds of water = a reduction of 8 pounds, 75 percent being water. Such excessive fluid elimination can lead to dehydration that further impedes the true fat-metabolizing process.

- → Any fat loss that may occur from a low-carbohydrate diet results from caloric reduction and not from the absence of carbohydrates.

→ The lost water weight is quickly regained once eating returns to normal and the glucose/glycogen stores are replenished.

→ There is no hard scientific evidence to support the notion that the source of the calorie—not the calorie itself—is the key factor in becoming leaner. Gorging on dietary fat and protein instead of carbs will only cause the body to accumulate more stored fat.

→ Lack of carbohydrate, combined with an emphasis on fat and protein, leads to an unhealthy condition called ketosis. Besides producing bad breath, ketosis causes the body to pull nutrients from its muscles, heart, and other internal organs.

→ The high dietary-fat content of most low-carbohydrate diets is harmful to the cardiovascular system.

→ Without significant carbohydrates—in the form of fruits, vegetables, and whole grains—the diet predisposes users to a long-term risk of cancer.

→ A high-protein diet is especially risky for patients with diabetes because it can speed kidney disease.

→ Daily living without significant amounts of dietary carbohydrates is not conducive to an active lifestyle. And it deprives the brain of its primary source of fuel, thus contributing to a feeling of fatigue, "brain fog," and even depression.

→ Most overweight people rarely endure strict low-carbohydrate dieting on their own for longer than 2 weeks. The initial weight loss from the elimination of water, however, gives them a false sense of success. Many believe that if they had continued longer, they would have reached their goal. Thus, the low-carbohydrate eating practices appear to work when in fact they don't, and these beliefs continue to be reinforced.

Carbohydrates and Maintenance

According to a study reported in a 1998 edition of the *Journal of the American Dietetic Association,* people who successfully lost an average of 30 pounds and kept them off for 5 years did so by eating more, not less, carbohydrate.

On the one hand, there are some carbohydrate-rich foods—such as candies, baked goods, and regular soft drinks—that should be limited on a fat-loss diet. On the other hand, as most registered dietitians proclaim, any carbohydrate-rich food has a place on a reducing diet, if it's consumed in moderation with a variety of other nutrients. Actually, both sides have merit.

I believe that a variety of carbohydrate-rich foods is essential for successful fat loss as well as maintenance. And these foods are a key energy provider for productive negative-accentuated training, which is the catalyst in the entire fat-loss process.

FAT LOSS AND HANGING SKIN

SOME PEOPLE WHO LOSE SIGNIFICANT POUNDS of fat sometimes end up with a layer of hanging skin, which is usually at the front or sides of the waist. Age plays a role, as people in their twenties and thirties have more elasticity in their skin, as opposed to people in their fifties and sixties. Also, some people have inherited characteristics of the skin that make them more prone to hanging skin.

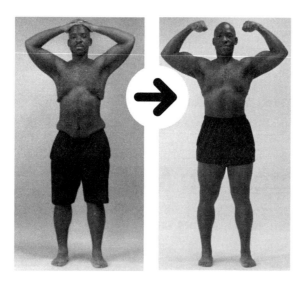

Clifton Powell, 26, started the Breakthrough program at a height of 5 feet 10 inches and a weight of 208.5 pounds. After 6 weeks, he lost 24.28 pounds of fat and 5 inches off his waist. He also built 10.53 pounds of muscle, which helped him shrink some of his loose skin.

Combating Holiday Calories

It seems that there's a major holiday in almost each month of the year. As a result, you'll be eating and drinking more often at locations out of your direct control. Here are four defensive steps to take:

→ **Plan ahead, eat ahead.** If the festivity includes dinner, find out what is on the menu. If there are not enough good choices or dinner is served

Clifton Powell, pictured opposite, was a fascinating participant who had an issue with hanging skin. Clifton had lost 56 pounds during the preceding year on a lower-calorie diet of his own design. During that time, he did no strength training. His before photo revealed several inches of hanging skin over the sides of his chest and waist.

During the Body Fat Breakthrough program, Clifton trained intensely and followed the eating and water-drinking schedule consistently for 6 weeks. His hanging skin shrank significantly. His muscularity also improved dramatically, as he built 10.53 pounds of muscle and added 0.5 inch to each upper arm.

I tell all my trainees who have significant amounts of hanging skin to be patient, to let time do its work. Often it takes 12 months for the skin to adapt to a successful trainee's new size and shape.

After a year, if the skin is still hanging, then the idea is to simply deal with it by wearing the appropriate clothing. A still-frustrated individual, as a last resort, may want to consult with a plastic surgeon.

Surgery is the only way to remove the skin permanently, but that doesn't mean it's right for most people. It involves general anesthesia, suturing, recovery, and scarring. And it's costly, and most patients have to pay out of pocket, as insurance rarely covers cosmetic surgery.

My best advice is to get the fat off, keep building your muscles, continue to stay hydrated, dress appropriately, and be patient.

well past your normal mealtime, eat at home. Budget 100 to 200 calories for some polite eating at the party.

→ **Limit alcohol intake.** Alcohol is one of the most calorie-dense foods. Alcohol also tends to be accompanied by high-calorie snacking. As judgment blurs, there's more to drink and more to eat. Social drinking can produce a quantum leap in your daily calories. Couldn't you still enjoy your party if you halved your alcohol intake? Never drink alcohol when you're thirsty. Quench your thirst with water. If you are having mixed drinks, drink the mixer every other round.

→ **Say no firmly but gracefully.** You'll flatter the hostess—and avoid eating her megacalorie offering—by telling her how delicious the dish looks and requesting the recipe. But explain that you're unable to eat it right now. You must be firm. This won't be easy, because others will tempt you and even resent you. Tell them you have to fit into a new pair of jeans, or offer a similar reason.

→ **Cut calories when not at social functions.** During the most tempting festive seasons, trim a moderate amount from your daily breakfast, lunch, and dinner. Never drop below 250 calories a meal. And never skip meals.

Eating Out on the Body Fat Breakthrough Plan

In today's health-and-fitness-conscious society, virtually no restaurant is going to be surprised by or unprepared to accommodate special dietary requests. The problem is not with them but with knowing how to explain what you want. Here are the best ways to order a suitable meal:

→ **Request that a large pitcher of ice water be placed on your table.** Drink freely before, during, and after the meal.

→ **Leave the menu unopened.** The purpose of the menu is to entice you to spend big, and restaurants really know how to sell the sizzle.

→ **Choose a simple green salad without garnishes such as croutons and bacon bits.** Lemon juice, vinegar, or a low-calorie preparation is preferable to any creamy or oily dressing.

- **Select one or two vegetables with nothing added.** A plain baked potato is nearly always available. Other good choices are broccoli, cauliflower, and carrots.

- **Ask the waiter what kind of fresh fish is available.** Order a whitefish and have it baked, broiled, or steamed with nothing on it. Although chicken is acceptable, it is usually prepared earlier in the day with certain types of added marinades—which mean extra calories.

- **Be very specific with your order.** Double-check to make certain that your waiter understands exactly what you want. Don't be afraid to send something back to the kitchen if it's not what you requested.

- **Have coffee or tea for dessert** or, at most, some fresh strawberries or raspberries.

- **Reinforce the waiter and the manager as you leave.** Make them aware of your specific likes and dislikes about the food and the service.

Eating while on Vacation

Vacations can be relaxing or stressful, depending on your planning, preparation, and finances. Here are a few more hints to assist you in keeping your dietary calories under control:

- **Avoid calorie-dense foods.** Load up on foods such as salads, vegetables, and broiled fish. (See the guidelines above.)

- **Plan ahead.** Have plenty of healthy snacks available during the day.

- **Fill a big pitcher with ice water.** Cool yourself by drinking plenty of water instead of having high-calorie sodas or ice cream.

- **Apply an activity-oriented plan.** Biking, hiking, boating, and mountain climbing are calorie-burning activities that relax and refresh the mind.

- **Sweat right.** Don't mistake the dehydration of sunbathing for activity. Just because you perspire doesn't mean you're burning significant calories.

→ **Maintain your fitness schedule.** Set exercise goals for your vacation. Most fitness centers will sell you a pass for a day or a week.

→ **Avoid happy hour.** Drink alcohol sparingly, if at all.

→ **Keep your mind engaged.** Read at least one inspiring book—perhaps fitness oriented?

Add Aromas and Textures

Many people are attracted to a simple, basic, easy-to-prepare eating plan. As a result, I've tried to keep the Breakthrough plan diet primarily plain vanilla. I also realize, however, that there are individuals who enjoy experimenting with various seasonings and ingredients that can add some pizzazz to "diet" foods that have a reduced level of calories, fat, and salt.

An interesting way to add creativity to basic meals is through food ingredients that are rich in fragrant aromas, vibrant colors, and varied textures. A listing of some of these ingredients, as well as a few practical examples, follows:

→ Freshly ground allspice makes a terrific accent when it is scattered over freshly cooked greens, carrots, or beans.

→ Dijon mustard can be used in place of mayonnaise on any sandwich. This great-tasting mustard, which has only 4 calories per teaspoon, combines well with canned tuna.

→ Bell peppers come in yellow, red, and green varieties. Their mild, crisp sweetness can add sparkle to any salad. When roasted, they can be used to garnish pasta, fish, and poultry.

→ Red cabbage, which is actually purple, may be finely shredded and added raw to meals that need color and crispness.

→ Bean sprouts in several varieties are now available in many supermarkets. They have a fresh, clean taste and texture, which perks up sandwiches of all types.

→ Radishes provide unique crispness and bite. Their tart taste and texture will blend with the most delicate flavors in salads and sauces.

These examples are low in calories and high in aroma, color, or texture. You may use them freely throughout the Breakthrough menus.

Find a Partner for Problems

Having a partner progress through the Body Fat Breakthrough program with you is a step in the right direction for most people. Your partner—whether a spouse, friend, coworker, or neighbor—should be someone you can talk to about your goals, your meals, and your workouts. Make a plan to talk (or e-mail) 5 minutes every day.

Although not always possible, the ideal partner is someone who is progressing through the program with you. Share this book, trade small talk, contribute experiences, and enjoy triumphs together.

What's better than experiencing the satisfaction of achieving your goal? Helping someone else do the same.

Backslide Forward

You may have adhered to the Body Fat Breakthrough diet strictly for weeks. Then, one day, the scent of fresh-from-the-oven cinnamon buns pulls you into a doughnut shop. Fifteen minutes later, you've wolfed down two big, cream-filled buns!

You may be progressing nicely with your negative-accentuated routine. An unexpected emergency, however, causes you to miss two workouts.

Now you feel guilty. You broke the diet. You slacked off on your exercise. You feel like you might as well forget the entire program and go back to your old ways.

Don't let yourself fall into this senseless, destructive trap. Guilt saps your motivation and confidence.

Furthermore, such thinking indicates only a short-term goal. True power revolves around the realization that permanent fat loss is a long-term project that is bound to have ups and downs.

Expect to backslide occasionally. You're only human, right? There is no disgrace in backsliding. The disgrace lies in letting a lapse get you so discouraged that you quit trying. You must keep moving forward.

JACK WILLIS
BEFORE & AFTER

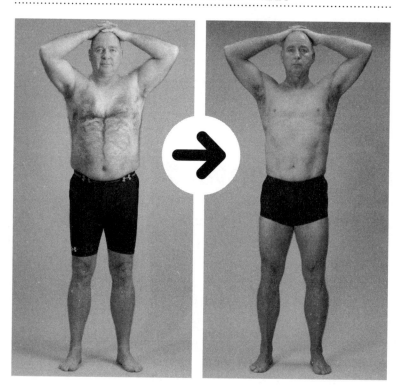

AGE 53, HEIGHT 5'10"

BEFORE BODY WEIGHT

212
POUNDS

AFTER BODY WEIGHT

179
POUNDS

AFTER 18 WEEKS

38.11
POUNDS OF FAT LOSS

9
INCHES OFF WAIST

5.11
POUNDS OF MUSCLE GAIN

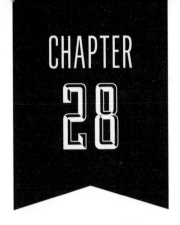

CHAPTER

28

FAT BOMB #9:
Realistic Evaluations

Check your progress and boost your motivation to keep going strong

FOR the past 6 weeks you've been losing fat and building muscle. If you've applied yourself, according to the instructions in this book, you should definitely be seeing and feeling some big differences.

To determine your specific results, turn back to Chapter 24 and retake all your measurements. When you're finished, you'll want to compare your results with the average expectations for men or for women.

Win by Losing and Building

In 2012 at Gainesville Health & Fitness, I worked with 41 men and 77 women who progressed through my 6-week Body Fat Breakthrough program. I

GENDER, HEIGHT, AND FAT LOSS

GENDER AND HEIGHT PLAY IMPORTANT ROLES in fat loss. On similar eating and exercising plans, men lose significantly more fat than do women. The primary reason is that men, compared with women, have more muscle mass and, consequently, higher metabolisms. Taller participants also have an advantage over shorter ones because they have more skin available to the environment, which allows for greater heat/calorie/fat transfer.

Note the heights of these selected trainees and their individual fat losses after the first 2 weeks (below).

If you are a shorter, overweight female, do not get discouraged. The same principles that work so well for taller men and women will still work for you. It will simply take more time for you to reach your goal.

There is also an occasional exception to the above rules. Turn back to

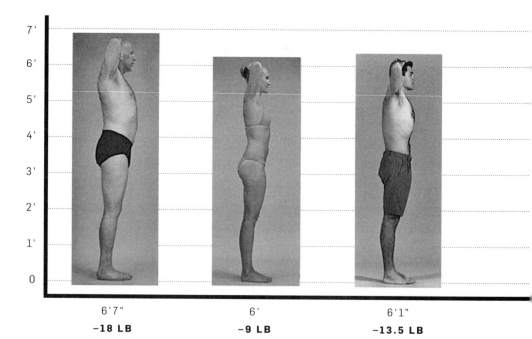

6'7"	6'	6'1"
−18 LB	**−9 LB**	**−13.5 LB**

selected these 118 people for the study not only because they were overfat and out of shape but also because they were all highly motivated.

I pushed each subject through the negative-accentuated workout and monitored him or her carefully through daily e-mails. I encouraged each subject

Chapter 21, page 199, and look at the before-and-after photos of Melissa Norman. Because of her height—5-foot-2—I tried to talk her out of signing up for my initial Breakthrough group. She told me she absolutely could not be talked into quitting before she started, nor would she quit at the end of 6 weeks or 12 weeks. Then she looked me in the eyes with old-school determination and said she wanted to commit for the long haul. With that kind of fervor, she received my okay. During the following 2 weeks, Melissa lost 10.5 pounds of fat—which was the best of any woman.

Melissa Norman was not only an exception to the rules but, as a participant, she was *exceptional*—exceptional in her motivation, discipline, and follow-through. Of the 77 women who finished my Breakthrough program in 2012, she finished in the number one position in overall fat loss.

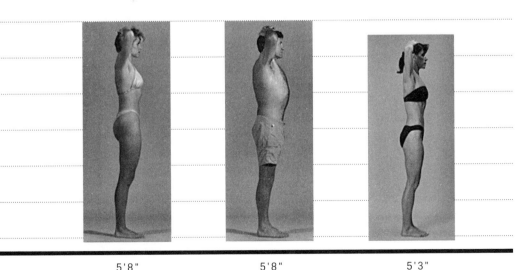

5'8"
−6 LB

5'8"
−8.5 LB

5'3"
−2.5 LB

to do the cold plunge after a workout and walk after evening meals. We held group meetings at the end of each 2-week period, at which questions were answered and concepts were discussed.

My test panel subjects had an advantage over you in that they were pushed, monitored, encouraged, and made accountable to an experienced coach during the entire 6 weeks. As a result, the average pounds and inches lost by these men and women were above what I expect your results will be. Still, your results should be significant—about 80 to 90 percent of the results of the GHF groups. Below you'll find the results of the test panel, followed by figures representing 80 to 90 percent of those numbers, shown in bold, for each gender.

	GAINESVILLE MEN	MEN YOUR EXPECTED RESULTS	GAINESVILLE WOMEN	WOMEN YOUR EXPECTED RESULTS
FAT LOSS IN POUNDS	27.5	22–24.75	15.5	12.4–13.95
INCHES OFF WAIST	5.1	4.1–4.6	4	3.2–3.6
MUSCLE GAIN IN POUNDS	8	6.4–7.2	4.6	3.68–4.14

If you accurately measured your body weight and percent body fat before and after the 6-week program, your improvement should be near these numbers.

Furthermore, if you took whole-body pictures of yourself in a bathing suit 6 weeks ago, you'll want to take them again. You should be able to see definite improvement when you compare your before and after photographs side by side. For valid comparisons, be sure to make your height in both sets of pictures exactly the same. Of course, many of you will exceed both the fat-loss and muscle-gain numbers. And you should be able to see your overall results throughout your body in your before and after photo comparisons.

My most successful fat-loss group was the very first one. The participants average results are listed in Chapter 6. If you exceeded the averages for the Gainesville men or Gainesville women, compare your results to those in Group 1 in Chapter 6.

The Next Step

Have you reached some or all of your goals that you established during the past 6 weeks? Are you satisfied or dissatisfied with the way you look?

Maybe you lost 15, 20, or even 30 pounds of fat on my 6-week course, but you still have more pounds and inches to lose. It took you a little longer than 6 weeks to put it on, and it's going to take a while longer to get it off.

You probably have to weigh well over 250 pounds to lose 35 pounds of fat or more in 6 weeks. Yet Bob Smith, whom you met in Chapter 4, removed 54 pounds. Bob was 6 feet 7 inches tall and weighed 302 pounds when he started. So if you weigh less than 250 pounds and have more than 30 pounds of fat to eliminate, there's a high probability that it's going to require longer than 6 weeks. If you're in this category, here's what to do.

1. MAKE ANOTHER COMMITMENT

Decide now that you want to continue. You've already taken some major steps toward removing your excess body fat and improving your health. You've made significant progress by sticking to the plan for 6 weeks. Make a commitment for another 6 weeks or less, if you believe you can reach your goal sooner.

Some individuals require three or four times, 18 to 24 weeks, before they reach their satisfaction level. Simply turn the week-by-week dieting, exercising, and other practices into week-by-week steps that move you closer and closer toward your goal.

2. TAKE A WEEK OFF

You may think I'm contradicting myself if I tell you to take a week off after I just asked you to make a commitment to further dieting and exercising. Most of the men and women who continued with the plan felt that a week off renewed their enthusiasm.

Be careful not to gorge yourself with food. You probably would have difficulty doing so even if you tried. Simply eat approximately 400 more calories per day than you were eating during weeks 5 and 6—or approximately 1,800 calories a day for a man and 1,600 calories a day for a woman. Keep drinking your water: 1 gallon a day.

After a week off, you'll be eager to repeat the 6-week course.

3. REPEAT THE DIET

Six weeks ago, in 2-week phases, you gradually decreased your calories—if you are a man—from 1,600 to 1,500 to 1,400 per day. A woman went from 1,400 to 1,300 to 1,200 per day. Now that you've added a few pounds of muscle to your body, you should be able to progress through the same descending-calorie plan with similar results. Again, start at 1,600 calories for men and 1,400 for women.

Furthermore, this time around you'll be more familiar with the menus and foods. You'll be able to gauge servings without actually weighing and measuring. The entire process will be easier. Just be sure your daily calories remain at the appropriate level.

You may be wondering why this down-up-down plan is recommended in preference to sticking to the same number of calories each day, week, and month. The down-up-down method is effective for three reasons:

→ Such a diet supplies you with needed variety.

→ Mixing up the status quo seems to benefit your body's fat-burning process.

→ When your calories go up, so does your energy level. Such an increase in energy level may be just the motivation you need to train harder and then stimulate additional muscle growth.

You can continue this down-up-down eating plan for as long as 12 months, or until you attain your fat-loss goal.

4. ADD A LITTLE TUNA

Interestingly, Angel Rodriguez and Melissa Norman, the man and woman who lost the most fat in Gainesville, both progressed through the Breakthrough program six consecutive times. And both of them ate the tuna salad recipe that I provide on page 240 several times each week. Here are a few more favorite tuna recipes.

Tuna-Pineapple Combo (255)

In a large bowl, mix the following:

$\frac{1}{2}$ can (2.5 ounces) chunk light tuna in water, drained (50)

$\frac{1}{4}$ cup (2 ounces) dark red kidney beans (65)

$^1\!/_2$ cup (4 ounces) pineapple chunks, water packed (50)

2 tablespoons sweet relish (40)

1 tablespoon Hellmann's Light Mayonnaise (50)

Tuna-Bean Delight (280)

In a large bowl, mix the following:

$^1\!/_2$ can (2.5 ounces) chunk light tuna in water, drained (50)

$^1\!/_2$ cup (4 ounces) canned sweet peas (60)

$^1\!/_2$ cup (4 ounces) canned three-bean salad, drained (70)

$^1\!/_2$ apple (3" diameter), chopped (50)

1 tablespoon Hellmann's Light Mayonnaise (50)

Tuna-Chicken Vegetable Blitz (270)

In a large bowl, mix the following:

$^1\!/_2$ can (2.5 ounces) chunk light tuna in water, drained (50)

$^1\!/_2$ cup (4 ounces) Campbell's Healthy Request Condensed Soup, Chicken Vegetable (do not add water) (80)

$^1\!/_2$ cup (4 ounces) whole-kernel corn, canned, no salt added (60)

$^1\!/_2$ ounce dry-roasted peanuts (80)

Feel free to substitute any of the above for a Breakthrough dinner or lunch.

5. CONTINUE YOUR NEGATIVE-ACCENTUATED TRAINING

During the last 2 weeks of the 6-week program, you did one set of 10 exercises, and you performed them once a week. You should continue with this routine of 10 exercises once a week until you lose your excess fat. Don't do less or more than 10 exercises.

Your negative-accentuated goal is to double your strength in all your basic exercises. If you did 100 pounds on the chest press machine for 30-30-30 when you started, then your goal is to perform 200 pounds for 30-30-30. Many can reach that goal within 4 to 6 months on the basic exercises.

Once this goal is reached, you should modify your routine by adding some different exercises to your workout. The next chapter discusses how this is accomplished.

Your other practices—such as walking, superhydration, and extra sleeping—should remain unchanged from weeks 5 and 6.

6. CONCENTRATE ON INTELLIGENT ACTION.

➜ Patience is truly a virtue when it comes to losing those last few pounds.

➜ Hang in there. Those fat cells can shrink. Your dream, if it is realistic, can be achieved. It does take time, however.

➜ Be patient. Stick to the plan in this book. Take it 1 day at a time.

➜ Make intelligent action your ally.

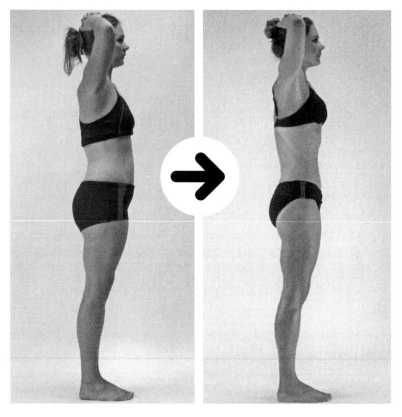

Julie McGinley transformed her body by trimming 4.75 inches off her waist, 4 inches off her hips, and 6 inches off her thighs.

FAT BOMB #9

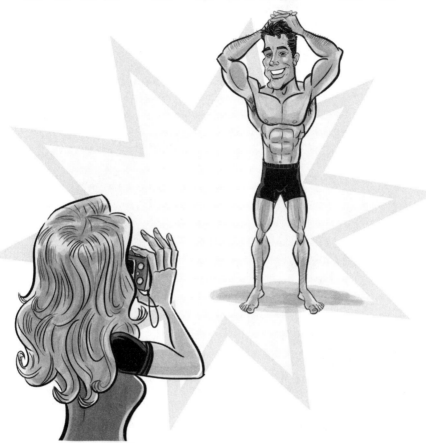

REALISTIC EVALUATIONS

Record, compare, and utilize before-and-after measurements and whole-body photgraphs of yourself in a tight-fitting bathing suit.

ANGEL RODRIGUEZ'S BODY TRANSFORMATION

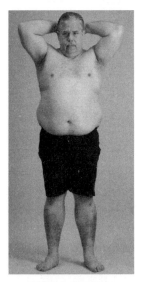

Before body weight:
281.5 pounds

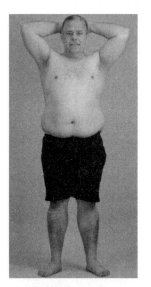

After 6 weeks:
250 pounds

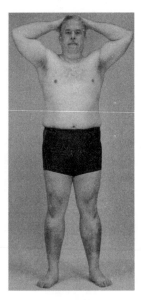

After 12 weeks:
223 pounds

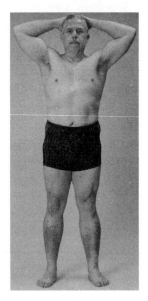

After 18 weeks:
204 pounds

THROUGH FIVE CONSECUTIVE 6-WEEK PROGRAMS

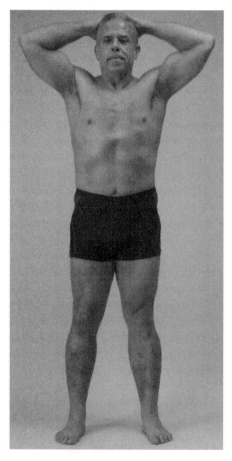

After 24 weeks:
190 pounds

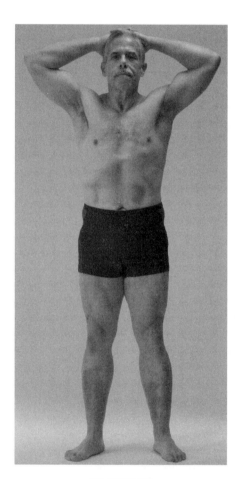

After 30 weeks:
181 pounds

Note: Angel Rodriguez's body weight went from 281.5 to 181, which was a reduction of 100.5 pounds. But he also gained 20.5 pounds of muscle. Thus, Angel's overall fat loss (weight loss + muscle gain) was 121 pounds.

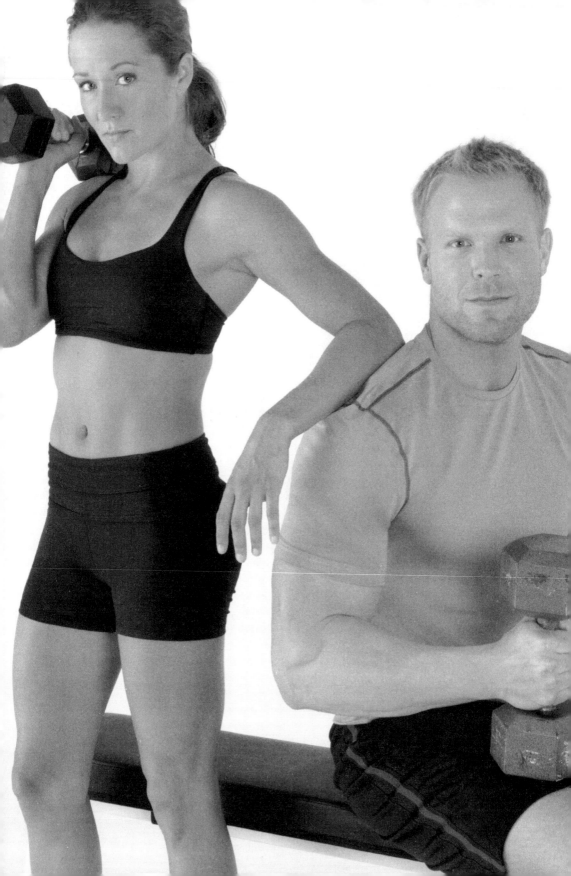

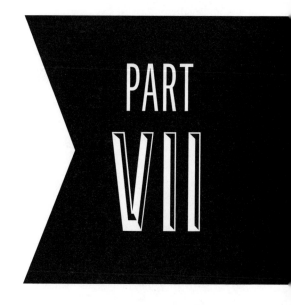

PART

VII

A Leaner, Stronger Body for Life

PHILIP SCHWARTZ
BEFORE & AFTER

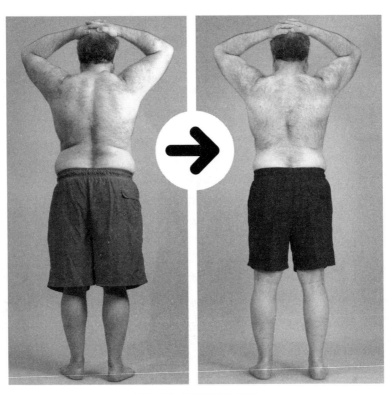

AGE 59, HEIGHT 5'7"

BEFORE BODY WEIGHT

229.25
POUNDS

AFTER BODY WEIGHT

196
POUNDS

AFTER 12 WEEKS

44.05
POUNDS OF FAT LOSS

8.75
INCHES OFF WAIST

10.8
POUNDS OF MUSCLE GAIN

CHAPTER 29

Guidelines for Keeping Your New Body

Sticking with the program for 100 days means adopting it for life!

ONCE you become satisfied with the condition of your body—whether it takes 6 weeks, 12 weeks, or 6 months—your next task is to maintain that status. Doing so requires certain adjustments to the guidelines and practices that you've been applying for the past several months. For this reason, this chapter on upkeep and preservation is one of the most important in the entire book.

Study the following adjustments.

1. ADHERE TO A CARBOHYDRATE-RICH, MODERATE-CALORIE EATING PLAN

Your eating plan is still carbohydrate rich, but you do not need to decrease the calories. You should now raise your calories to a moderate level. Instead of eating from 1,200 to 1,600 calories a day, consume from 1,800 to 2,400 a day. Maybe you can eat even more after your new body weight has stabilized.

There is no way to determine in advance how many calories you will need to maintain your new body weight. Trial-and-error experimentation will make the level obvious.

You should probably begin with 1,800 calories per day and see what happens after a week. If your body weight keeps going down, raise the calories to 1,900 or 2,000, depending on how much weight you lost during the week. Soon you should reach a level where your body weight stabilizes. This level is your daily calorie requirement.

Always keep your calories rich in carbohydrates. The 50-25-25 ratio of carbohydrates, proteins, and fats is not only ideal for losing fat but also appropriate for maintenance. Fruits, vegetables, breads, and cereals are your primary sources of carbohydrates. On your maintenance eating plan, strive each day to consume four servings of vegetables and fruits and four servings of breads and cereals. Doing so will allow your other foods—meats and dairy products—to fall into the correct ratio naturally.

2. EAT SMALLER MEALS MORE FREQUENTLY

You've been limiting each of your six meals per day to 400 calories or less. To maintain your body weight, set the limit per meal at 500 calories or less if you're a woman, or 600 calories or less if you're a man. A 500- to 600-calorie meal will still keep the insulin responses small. Furthermore, 500 to 600 calories is something you can easily adapt to—at least, most of the time.

What happens when you occasionally eat more than 500 or 600 calories at one time? Don't panic. Simply understand that you will sometimes backslide. Anticipate, plan, and get back on track.

3. DRINK 128 OUNCES OF COLD WATER EACH DAY

I hope by now you've seen and felt the benefits of drinking plenty of cold water. Make it a permanent part of your new lifestyle to consume 128 ounces, or 1 gallon, of water each day.

4. PERFORM NEGATIVE-ACCENTUATED EXERCISE ONCE A WEEK—OR LESS

You never outgrow your need for larger, stronger muscles. As you age, larger and stronger muscles become more and more important. Bigger muscles improve performance, add shape, stabilize joints, burn more calories, and allow you to live longer stronger.

There are four differences between your maintenance routines and your past workouts.

First, during maintenance, you can introduce more variety to your routine by adding some new exercises and removing some old ones. Some individuals in the Gainesville group, in fact, alternate standard strength-training workouts with negative-accentuated workouts. Standard strength-training routines are thoroughly covered in a previous book of mine titled *The New High-Intensity Training* (Rodale, 2004).

Second, with maintenance, you can reduce the number of exercises per routine slightly. Instead of doing one set of 10 exercises, try one set of seven or eight exercises. As your muscles get stronger, you actually need less strengthening exercise. For example, your workout might involve two lower-body exercises and five upper-body movements.

Third, some very strong individuals may want to experiment with reducing their frequency of training to one workout every 10 days. My good friend Jim Flanagan is one of the strongest men I know. In 2012, he trained only 36 times—which is a frequency that he considers ideal. And that ideal frequency is once every 10 days.

Fourth, with maintenance, you can add other forms of exercise—such as cardiovascular (Zumba, dancing, Spinning, or swimming) or sports (tennis, golf, basketball, or running) back into your weekly lifestyle.

5. WALK AFTER YOUR EVENING MEAL

Walking with food in your stomach is a good way to relax and burn extra calories. Although it's not necessary to do every day of the week, you should still take advantage of this effect often during your maintenance plan.

6. SLEEP AN EXTRA HOUR EACH NIGHT

Extra sleep is like extra water: You didn't know what you were missing until you tried it. It will be to your advantage to maintain your sleeping schedule every night you can.

7. APPLY OTHER FAT-LOSS PRACTICES

You may apply the fat-loss practices from Part V anytime they are needed during your maintenance program. With an understanding of these concepts, your arsenal should remain well stocked.

Internalize for Success

Over the years, I've trained thousands of people to build muscle and lose weight. Those who kept the fat off have done so because of internalization. The salient rules—for example, eat smaller meals, superhydrate your system, keep your muscles strong—have been internalized. "Internalizing" simply means making an action rote or automatic.

How long does it take to internalize? Behavioral psychologists say that it

WHAT WE CAN LEARN FROM COACH BOB KNIGHT

WHEN I WAS GROWING UP IN TEXAS, I played a lot of football and basketball. All my best coaches were former military men who believed in hard-nosed discipline, telling their athletes what *not* to do, and punishment for continued mistakes. When Bob Knight achieved notoriety coaching basketball at Indiana University during the 1970s, I was attracted to his tough techniques and out-spoken behaviors.

I've never met Bob Knight, but I feel like I know him. He's been interviewed numerous times on television, and he's frequently a guest commentator as part of ESPN's basketball coverage. Knight never hesitates to "tell it like he sees it," which usually involves listing of mistakes and more mistakes.

Knight's 2013 book, *The Power of Negative Thinking*, with its creative title, was a meaningful study for me. In fact, what he says about winning an important game has direct application to fat-off maintenance. In his book, Knight advises that after winning a big game, you should get over it quickly, because a happy moment can keep you from preparing adequately for the next opponent.

Winning one game does not make a season. Success is not short term.

takes 21 days to establish a pattern and 100 days to make it automatic.

I've observed similar time spans among my group participants. The Body Fat Breakthrough gets easier for most individuals after 3 weeks. If they stick with the discipline for 3 months, their daily behaviors adapt and become almost automatic. I believe there's power in 100 days. These 100-day men and 100-day women have a higher probability of keeping off their lost fat permanently.

You might say that automatic behavior in eating and exercising requires 100 days. But is that truly automatic? With some individuals, yes. With others, no. My experience in working with thousands of men and women shows that 200 days of practice is better than 100. Within reason, more is better.

Practice and more practice of proper eating and exercise is the key to losing fat. More important, because you are building a strong shield against the temptation to return to your old ways of coping, more compliance is the key to making sure your lost fat stays off for good.

Success is a long, enduring grind. Success is operating at a high level, with minimal mistakes, on a consistent basis.

If Bob Knight was speaking to my graduating class of Body Fat Breakthrough participants or to you, he might say:

Okay, I know many of you have lost 30 to 40 pounds of fat, and some of you even 90 to 100 pounds or more of fat. Big deal! Call your Aunt Polly and tell her about it. The real work—keeping it off—is just beginning. If you want to celebrate what you've achieved, keep your lost fat off for the next 1,825 days. That's 5 years. Take a look at the calendar and circle this date. I'll be back . . . and ready to party with you in early 2019. Wipe that cake and smile off your faces and start preparing for next year and the year after . . . right now.

Bob Knight is correct. Preparing beats repairing. Good preparation and planning, along with healthy negative thinking, is always the best approach, rather than going forward with carried-away zeal.

Thank you, Coach Knight, for forcing us to remove our rose-colored glasses.

JENNIFER STANSFIELD
BEFORE & AFTER

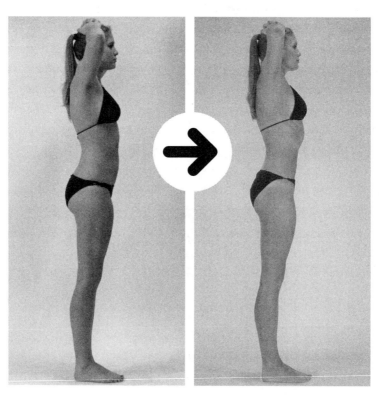

AGE 20, HEIGHT 5'7"

BEFORE BODY WEIGHT

131.2
POUNDS

AFTER BODY WEIGHT

119.8
POUNDS

AFTER 6 WEEKS

17.8
POUNDS OF FAT LOSS

4.625
INCHES OFF WAIST

6.4
POUNDS OF MUSCLE GAIN

CHAPTER

30

All Your Questions Answered

What you need to know about headaches, warmups, CrossFit, and more

THE following questions and answers should help fill in any remaining gaps about the Body Fat Breakthrough plan. These are among the most frequently asked questions among the individuals participating in my test-panel programs.

Running for Walking

Q: ***What about substituting running for the daily walk?***
A: *No, running is too vigorous an activity. You could also easily upset your stomach if you try to run immediately after your evening meal. The idea is to turn up your body heat without upsetting your digestion. Walking is the best choice.*

Headaches

Q: I often get headaches when I eat 1,200 calories a day. What should I do?

A: *Perhaps going longer than 3 hours between meals or snacks causes your headaches. If so, try spacing your eating episodes closer together.*

Also, some people who normally drink regular coffee with caffeine get headaches when they cut back or eliminate coffee. I'm okay with you having two cups of coffee or tea with caffeine in the morning.

Q: I got a bad headache from doing the negative-accentuated squat. How do I deal with it?

A: *Instead of doing the squat first, do it last. That should eliminate the problem.*

Q: Sometimes I get a headache when I drink ice-cold water. Can I drink the water without it being chilled?

A: *Yes, but you won't get the 123-calories-per-gallon thermogenic effect from warming the cold water to core body temperature. Try drinking the water more gradually (sipping with a large straw is best). You may have been consuming it too rapidly.*

Lunch for Dinner and Substitutions

Q: May I have my dinner for lunch and my lunch for dinner?

A: *Yes.*

Q: For breakfast, can I substitute a fresh bagel from my local deli for the recommended store-bought variety?

A: *No, unless the calories are the same. Unfortunately, most deli bagels contain from 50 to 100 percent more calories than the allowed-for 240 calories.*

Warming Up

Q: What about warming up before my negative-accentuated routine?

A: I do not believe that an elaborate warmup is desirable before a negative-accentuated routine. But I don't object to a few smooth, calisthenic movements—such as arm circles, trunk twists, and leg shakes—performed beforehand as a general warmup. In the recommended negative-accentuated routine, specific warming up of each body part occurs during the first 30 seconds of each exercise.

Cooling down after your workout prevents blood from pooling in your more recently worked muscles. After your final exercise, cool down by walking around the exercise area, getting a drink of water, and moving your arms in slow circles. Continue these easy movements for 4 or 5 minutes, or until your breathing rate returns to normal.

Bruises on Thighs

Q: I'm a 40-year-old woman who gets black and blue marks on my legs when I diet. Am I doing something wrong?

A: I don't believe you are doing anything wrong. Such black and blue marks are usually the result of increased estrogen circulating in your body, which weakens the walls of the capillaries and causes them to break under the slightest pressure. When this happens, blood escapes and a bruise occurs. Estrogen is broken down in the liver, and so is fat. When you are dieting, your liver breaks down the fat, leaving a lot more estrogen in the bloodstream.

It may be helpful to supplement your diet with a little extra vitamin C—100 milligrams per day—to help toughen the walls of the capillaries.

Vegetarian Meals

Q: Can a vegetarian follow your eating plan?

A: *Yes. Several vegetarians were among the 145 participants in Gainesville. Jeremy Leon, on page 250, in fact finished first in his group of 20 subjects. He lost more than 58 pounds of fat in 18 weeks. His favorite cookbook is* Vegetarian Cooking for Everyone *by Deborah Madison. The vegetarians that I've worked with over the past 3 decades have all been knowledgeable in the food and nutrition area. Here are some ways that they adapt the basic menus:*

➜ Sandwiches and salads: Instead of meat, use tofu or black beans.

➜ Soup: Instead of Healthy Choice Chicken & Dumplings, try Healthy Choice Garden Vegetable.

➜ Frozen microwaveable meals: The manufacturers that I recommend have Web sites that list vegetarian offerings. See Michelinas.com, Healthychoice.com, and Leancuisine.com.

CrossFit

Q: Should I do some of the CrossFit routines on my off days to burn some extra calories?

A: *CrossFit is a fitness company that provides vigorous exercise routines for more than 5,000 affiliated gyms throughout the United States. The problem with the CrossFit exercises is that every one of the recommended movements must be performed in a fast, ballistic manner. For example, you might be asked to do as many pushups as possible in 60 seconds, which are then followed by as many box jumps as possible in 60 seconds, and, finally, as many situps as you can do in another 60 seconds.*

From there, you might go to kettlebell curls, jumping rope, and burpees—each performed for another 60 seconds—and then to a rope climb, back extensions, and a fast walk with heavy kettlebells.

Certainly, once you learn to perform the various exercises correctly, with the proper resistance and repetitions, you can get a good overall workout. But you can also injure yourself, especially if you are in your forties or fifties and lack experience. You'll remember that all my recommended negative-accentuated movements are always performed smoothly—and not in a fast, ballistic fashion.

Some health-care professionals—and I'm one of them—note that the risk of injury from some CrossFit exercises outweighs their benefits, especially when they are performed with poor form in timed cycles.

To answer your question directly: No, I do not want you to burn extra calories with CrossFit. Any vigorous group of movements added to the Breakthrough program will eventually retard your fat loss.

Grams of Fat Per Day

Q: *How many grams of fat should I eat each day?*
A: *Men involved in the Breakthrough program average 1,500 calories per day and approximately 40 grams of fat over 6 weeks. Women average 1,300 calories and 35 grams of fat per day on the 6-week program.*

While you can certainly get too much fat from the food you eat, you can also get too little. A few women in our program were guilty of trying to cut too much fat. Thirty-five to 40 grams of fat per day works well for fat loss, nutritional well-being, and meal satisfaction.

Hormonally Speaking

Q: *I'm working on a PhD at the University of Florida, and I'm intrigued but also confused by your thoughts on activating key hormones through eccentric training. Can you help me better understand the hormone interactions?*
A: *I understand your confusion. Hormones are indeed a complex area. David Ponsonby, a researcher in Dallas, and Max Medary, MD, a neurosurgeon in Orlando, helped me organize my beliefs as follows:*

From a review of the scientific literature, combined with my studies in Gainesville, I believe the correct application of negative-accentuated training makes a deeper inroad into a person's starting level of strength. My research shows that this deeper inroad influences at least six hormones this way:

→ Stimulates growth hormone (GH) from the pituitary gland, which up-regulates the production of both IGF-1 and MGF. GH also facilitates the use of fat as fuel.

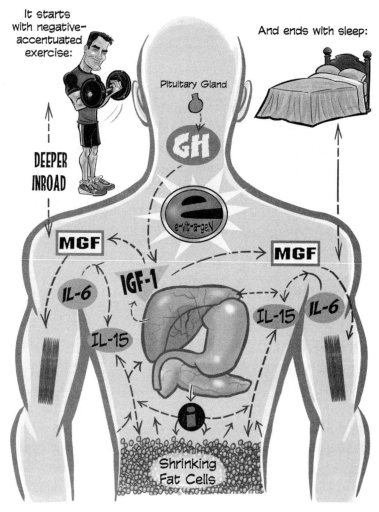

NEGATIVE TRAINING AND HORMONES:
How They Build Muscle and Shrink Fat

It starts with negative-accentuated exercise:

DEEPER INROAD

Pituitary Gland

GH

e-vit-a-geN

MGF

MGF

IGF-1

IL-6

IL-15

IL-15

IL-6

And ends with sleep:

Shrinking Fat Cells

- → Activates insulin-like growth factor (IGF-1), which is released by the liver and is relevant to muscle adaptation
- → Targets mechano-growth factor (MGF), which kick-starts the muscle-hypertrophy process
- → Mobilizes interleukin 6 (IL-6) within muscle, where it merges into the blood to help compensate for inflammation from training
- → Triggers interleukin 15 (IL-15), which encourages muscle/fat cross talk and promotes building muscle and metabolizing fat simultaneously
- → Directs the anabolic effects of insulin (i) from the pancreas on both fat and muscle

Negative training, by inciting the body's natural hormones, provides an important new way to lose fat and build muscle rapidly. This is the most cutting-edge advancement I've applied in 50 years of combating obesity.

I suspect that negative-accentuated training and its much deeper inroad brings into action a previously unknown hormone, a hormone that coordinates, unites, and enhances the six above into a championship team. I'm calling this unknown hormone e-vit-a-geN (that's *Negative* spelled backward) and I'm declaring that e-vit-a-geN orchestrates these skills from a central location in the upper body (see the drawing opposite).

Called upon once a week, e-vit-a-geN (e) and the other hormones—with the help of food, water, rest, and sleep—team to burn fat, build muscle, and reshape the body into the lean, strong machine that it was originally designed to become.

Extending the Walk

Q: *Will I get better fat-loss results if I extend the daily walk past the recommended 30 minutes?*

A: *Thirty minutes was chosen because it does not deplete significant amounts of your recovery ability. Remember, your body must be well rested to provide all the chemicals necessary for maximum fat loss and maximum muscle gain to occur. It's easily possible on a reduced-calorie diet, if you're not careful, to start burning the candle at both ends. Do not walk more than the recommended 30 minutes each day.*

30-30-30 Method

Q: *The negative-accentuated 30-30-30 method seems almost too easy if I try it with 80 percent of what I use for 8 to 12 repetitions. Should I add more resistance?*

A: *For some people, it may be too easy. Add resistance until it becomes more challenging.*

Q: *My positive movements on the 30-30-30 method are herky-jerky. Is that good or bad?*

A: *Some trainees have a tendency at first to move in a herky-jerky style, which is certainly not the best form. Keep trying and practice your focus. After a couple more sessions, your movements should become smoother and more fluid.*

Q: *What if I shorten the 30-30-30 style to 15-15-15 and double the reps?*

A: *I've tried that, and it doesn't work as well at stimulating the muscles involved. Stick with the 20- to 30-second phases on each of the three segments.*

Regular HIT for 30-30-30

Q: *Dr. Darden, I've followed your career and your recommended training plans for more than 20 years. For me 30-30-30 is not too easy—it's too difficult. Can I substitute your 3-second positive and 3-second negative style for 8 to 12 repetitions—which you describe in your book* The New High-Intensity Training—*for the 30-30-30 method, and then follow the rest of the Breakthrough program as you present it here?*

A: *Of the 10 factors, or Fat Bombs, that make up the success of this program, the one that's most responsible for the use of "Breakthrough" in* the title is X-Force training, or its stand-in, the 30-30-30 method. It's that important. Having said that, I hope you will reconsider and give 30-30-30 a fair trial.

On the other hand, here's a meaningful story from Gainesville.

During the Breakthrough selection process for Group 1, two women were disappointed that they did not get picked. Both of their husbands were selected. Without my knowledge, the women progressed through the first 6 weeks along with their husbands—with one exception: Instead of applying the negative-accentuated technique for each exercise of the strength-training routine, the two women substituted a similar exercise, which was then performed progressively for 8 to 12 repetitions.

What were their results? Over 6 weeks, each woman lost 12 pounds of body weight, which was about average for a woman who participated in one of my programs prior to the Breakthrough course.

And what were their husbands' results—in terms of weight, not fat? One lost 24 pounds and the other lost 28 pounds, which was an average of 26 pounds. Knowing the four people, as well as their starting body weights and other details, I would have expected the men to do 100 percent better than the women. But instead, they did 117 percent better, which was a 17 percent improvement over what I would have anticipated.

And now back to your question: Can you substitute one of my previous strength-training routines for this program's recommended 30-30-30 routine?

If you realize that the overall results are going to be less—less weight loss, less fat loss, and less muscle gain—then you can do that. But don't refer to what you're doing as my Body Fat Breakthrough program.

Power Athletes: How Much Protein Is Enough?

Q: *Some of the sports scientists at the University of Florida recommend extra protein intake for their strength and power athletes. Do you disagree with them, too?*

A: *I'm not against a little extra protein in your diet. Just don't go completely overboard and bump it up to three or four times the RDA. Consuming 250 to 300 grams of protein a day—whether it's from food or supplements—is expensive, wasteful, and not the safest thing you could do for your liver and kidneys.*

There has been research—including one study from the University of Florida—showing that perhaps there are advantages for power athletes and bodybuilders to consume from 50 to 100 percent more protein than the RDA of 0.36 gram of protein per pound of body weight. I don't buy into it—not completely, anyway.

Here's what I do believe about protein and muscle.

Only intense exercise generates cellular messages (hormones) that stimulate the chemicals to begin the process of expanding muscle fibers. An excess of dietary protein or any other nutrients won't generate these messages. Nutrition enters the picture only after the muscles are stimulated to grow. And even then, rest is at least as important as nutrition.

Muscle Magazines and Money

Q: Dr. Darden, what influenced you to consume so much protein earlier in your career?

A: *The same thing that influences bodybuilders today was what influenced me back in the 1960s. It was muscle magazines—10 years of reading almost every one published. These magazines all contained cleverly designed collections of editorials, articles, and advertisements that promoted protein supplements and high-protein eating.*

The facts show that you simply do not require much protein to build muscle. Human muscle is at least 70 percent water. Only 20 percent of muscle is protein. Because muscle is mostly water, 1 pound of muscle contains only 600 calories. Calories and water are more important to the muscle-building process than is protein.

But if you are the publisher of a leading bodybuilding magazine—from a promotional, money-making point of view—how much revenue could you produce from pushing calories and water? Calories and water are everywhere, at least in the United States. But as a sales pitch, "tasty calories and pure water" doesn't have the magic of the following phrases: "premium micro"; "ultrafiltration, whey protein"; "advanced protein synthesis complex"; "100% enzymatically digested bioactive protein isolate."

It doesn't matter what you call protein or how you promote the end result, the truth is that it's only minimally important to building muscle.

The most impressive bodybuilder that I've ever seen in my life, a man named Sergio Oliva, who had arms bigger than his head and who was the last bodybuilder to defeat Arnold Schwarzenegger in the Mr. Olympia contest, trained with Arthur Jones in Florida during the summer of 1971. Oliva trained extremely hard and sweated gallons as Jones pushed him in an unventilated Quonset hut with no air-conditioning. Each of their workouts resembled an episode from the TV drama The Walking Dead, *and I'm not kidding!*

What was Oliva's favorite after-workout dinner? A large pepperoni pizza, washed down with 32 ounces of Coca-Cola—not exactly a high-protein meal but more than adequate in calories and water.

Bodybuilding and Protein

Q: *I'm interested in bodybuilding. I'm sure you realize that just about everybody connected to bodybuilding says the opposite of what you say: They say that a high-protein diet is necessary for building large muscles. Are they all wrong in their beliefs?*

A: *Perhaps it's better to say that they all have been misled, badly misled. I've told this story about my experiences with protein in some of my bodybuilding books, and it's worth telling again.*

From 1970 to 1973, I studied nutrition at Florida State University with Harold Schendel, PhD, who had spent a number of years in Africa working with starving children. I remember him telling me about how his team of doctors rushed into a famine country, assembled the starving children, and tried to force-feed them high-protein diets. Rather than improve, their conditions got worse. They quickly realized that what these children needed were simple calories. What worked best was a mush mixture of water, sugar, and butter, with small amounts of protein, vitamins, and minerals.

Later in his career, Schendel had a hand in establishing the Recommended Dietary Allowance for protein. In 1970, he convinced me to do a 2-month study on my body to determine if massive protein intake was beneficial. Back then, because I was really into bodybuilding, I consumed more than 300 grams of protein a day.

I kept accurate records of my food intake and activity for 60 days, and I even collected my urine during the same period. Afterward, I used the Kjeldahl method for determining nitrogen in my urine, which is a measure of protein utilization.

To my surprise, anytime I consumed more than the RDA of protein, the excess was excreted in my urine. Schendel concluded that my kidneys were working overtime to metabolize the excess protein. He also explained that human kidneys and livers show overuse symptoms in the presence of massive amounts of protein. We know from long-term animal studies that high-protein diets will shorten life spans.

So I stopped my massive protein diet and immediately felt a surge of energy from unburdening my kidneys and liver. Over the next 2 years, on a carbohydrate-rich diet, I won several of the bodybuilding contests that I'd been trying so hard to win. Adding carbohydrates and subtracting proteins had made a significant difference in my appearance. As a result, I haven't consumed a high-protein diet since early 1970.

Say No! Think Simple!

Q: *Everything about losing fat and keeping it off seems so difficult. Can you help make it a little easier?*

A: *This book will be able to help you if you very carefully follow the advice that has worked so well for others. Every chapter in this book has been about how to simplify a complex situation.*

At the end of Chapter 1, I noted that the Body Fat Breakthrough program was not going to be easy. And then I commented that "nothing is meaningful if it's achieved easily."

In other words, "meaningful" and "easy" do not belong together.

If your goal is to get a leaner, stronger, and better-shaped body, you must practice and eventually master a number of salient steps. And each one of them, depending on your past experience, is relatively challenging. One helpful concept that you must apply repeatedly is the idea of saying no and meaning it. "No" gives you control.

At the end of Chapter 6, I pointed out that if you would stick with me and my program throughout this book, then I would help you make the process not easy, but simple.

You can accomplish your goals with the help of 10 Fat Bombs, which illustrate what to do in a straightforward manner. Adhere to these guidelines with the required discipline and patience and you'll be rewarded—rewarded with leanness, strength, and a better-shaped body—quickly in 6 to 12 weeks.

Get with the program.

Say no. Think simple.

That's my condensed version of losing fat and keeping it off.

BIGGER ARMS IN 2 WEEKS

BUILDING BIGGER ARMS IS THE SINGLE most popular topic among men interested in body development. It is also the subject matter that muscle magazines most often feature.

Among the hundreds of male bodybuilders at Gainesville Health & Fitness, I selected five for a special Bigger Arms in 2 Weeks course. Each man was trained twice a week on eight negative-accentuated exercises. The workout was finished in 15 minutes or less. Each man gave me his word that he would perform no other strength-training activity for 14 days.

The average muscle gain per man was 6.9 pounds, which was significant, since all of these men were advanced.

Edwin Brown, who goes by the nickname of Truck, topped the trainees, and his results were truly exceptional. Truck increased the size of each of his contracted upper arms by 0.625 inch. In the after photo of him on opposite page, his larger contracted arm, his left, measures 20.125 inches. That's right, I taped Truck's arm, in an unpumped cold condition, at slightly more than 20 inches in circumference.

A muscular, 20-inch arm is *big* almost beyond belief. You literally have to see it up close to believe it—and Truck Brown has one.

"All four negative-accentuated workouts pumped my arms like nothing before," Truck recalls. "I knew my biceps and triceps were going to grow, before they grew."

During the final measurements, 43-year-old Truck was 5 feet 10 inches tall and weighed 240 pounds. He had a 53.25-inch chest, a 34.75-inch waist, and 27-inch thighs. He has a truly impressive physique.

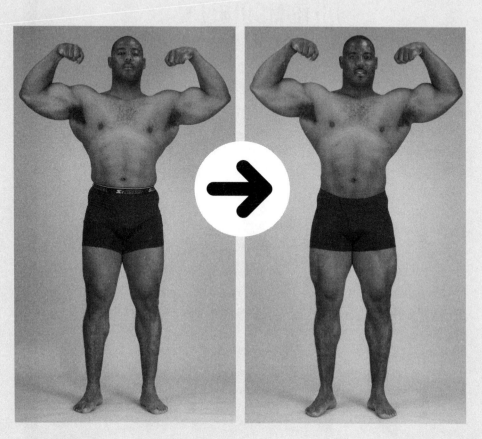

Edwin "Truck" Brown, from four brief negative-accentuated workouts spread over 2 weeks, built 12.71 pounds of muscle. He added 1.25 inches on his upper arms, 2.25 inches on his chest, and 2 inches on his thighs.

JULIE MCGINLEY
BEFORE & AFTER

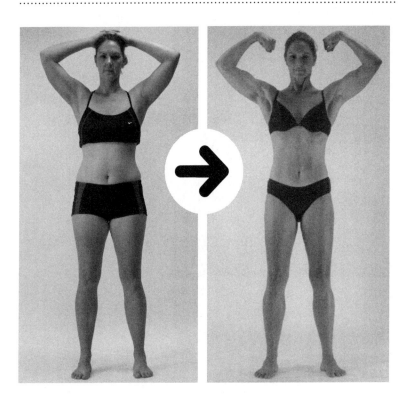

AGE 38, HEIGHT 5'7"

BEFORE BODY WEIGHT

160.5
POUNDS

AFTER BODY WEIGHT

143.5
POUNDS

AFTER 12 WEEKS

22.34
POUNDS OF FAT LOSS

4.75
INCHES OFF WAIST

5.34
POUNDS OF MUSCLE GAIN

FAT BOMB #10:
Overlearning

How to hang tough (and stay lean) for the rest of your life

METAPHORICALLY, you've reached the top of the mountain and figuratively left your own mountain of fat behind.

You have a new you to take care of now. Your biggest obstacle, especially in the early days, is not relapsing to your old body.

But exactly how do you stay lean and strong in a world where fast-food establishments monopolize every main street and prepared packages of food occupy every commercial break on television?

There's a rule that will help you with your long-term fat-loss management.

The Key to Consistency

In my home library, I probably have 200 books related to losing fat. About 185 of the books push diets that don't work; at least, they don't work over the long term. On the other hand, I have 14 books that are based on science, and they do work. The remaining book—one book out of 200—discusses keeping the lost fat off and keeping it off permanently.

The title of that book is *Keeping It Off: Winning at Weight Loss* by Drs. Robert H. Colvin and Susan C. Olson. While the book doesn't come out and name the concept, it's present in almost every chapter, and it is the key to not only sustaining your fat loss, but also to being consistent. I call that unnamed concept overlearning.

Overlearning means any practice that you do after you've already achieved a certain level of success. In scientific journals related to this subject, success is usually defined as an on-target trial. In other words, you're successful if, for example, you can toss a basketball into a net with your nondominant arm. You've already learned how to sink a basketball, but by overlearning through extended practice, you are able to do it consistently even though the challenge is more difficult. Researchers have studied the effects of practice beyond the point when the criterion learning has occurred and have come to the same conclusion: Overlearning results in better retention of material than regular learning.

No amount of practice seems enough for the serious-minded athlete. Larry Bird, the now-retired NBA basketball superstar, estimates that he shot the ball at the basket not thousands of times, not hundreds of thousands of times—but millions of times. Overlearning is one reason why Bird was such a superb basketball shooter.

The same thing can be said about today's NBA superstars, such as Kobe Bryant and LeBron James.

Is it any wonder that even after no practice, former college athletes can still demonstrate a high degree of proficiency in their areas of specialty? Of course, the average individual does not desire and perhaps lacks the ability to attain such a high level of skill. Although that person's time involvement will be considerably less than that of a college or professional athlete, it should be remembered that more practice of such fundamentals will increase the potential for almost any later-in-life skills.

What do successful athletes have in common with successful dieters? The answer, of course, is overlearning.

Overlearning and Fat Loss

Overlearning, as it relates to fat loss, involves the practice of certain behaviors again and again, until they are so ingrained that almost nothing can disturb them. Overlearning produces automatic-pilot actions. Without thinking, you demonstrate the correct behavioral response.

The more times you experience the desired response, the better you get and the more lasting the response. You gradually bypass your old response entirely, supplanting it with a new response and eliminating the transitional correction.

Throughout their book, Drs. Colvin and Olson interviewed dieters who had lost an average of 53.2 pounds and kept the fat off for an average of 6 years. After studying all the interviews, I came to the conclusion that the main ingredient for success was overlearning. All of the subjects followed a predictable pattern to permanent weight loss that they kept repeating daily, weekly, and monthly.

In spite of financial difficulties, lawsuits, divorce, life-threatening illnesses, serious accidents, and deaths of family and friends, they had not regained their lost fat. It was not because their lost weight was more important than such tragedies—far from it—but the habits required through practice were so deeply ingrained that theese dieters persisted even when stressful events came to the forefront.

Stay consistent by overlearning my 10 Fat Bombs (see page 305).

FAT BOMB #10

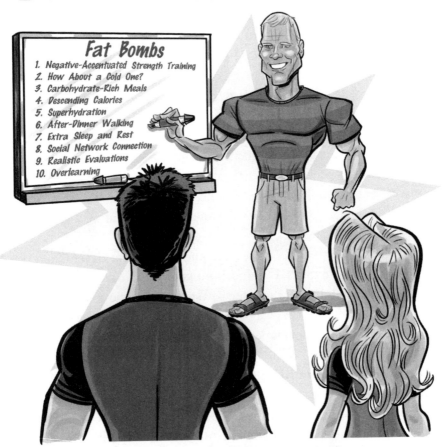

Fat Bombs
1. Negative-Accentuated Strength Training
2. How About a Cold One?
3. Carbohydrate-Rich Meals
4. Descending Calories
5. Superhydration
6. After-Dinner Walking
7. Extra Sleep and Rest
8. Social Network Connection
9. Realistic Evaluations
10. Overlearning

OVERLEARNING

The more you overlearn the FAT BOMBS, the higher the
probability is that your changes are permanent.

Making Mentors

It was July 21, 2013, and I was at a Gainesville Health & Fitness introductory meeting for another group of Body Fat Breakthrough participants. Lydia Maree, who was my top assistant during my 2012 research, had been running the program in Gainesville throughout 2013. She had successfully supervised 136 people through one or more of my 6-week programs in the first half of 2013. Earlier in the day, I helped Lydia measure and photograph a number of trainees who were finishing their third pass through the program. Some of the standouts:

→ Mark Vega, age 43, lost 87 pounds of fat and built 22 pounds of muscle.

→ Roger Crase, age 62, lost 45 pounds of fat and built 5 pounds of muscle.

→ Ryan Fisher, age 32, lost 19 pounds of fat and built 22 pounds of muscle. At a height of 6 feet 6 inches and a body weight of 230 pounds, Ryan could do well in a bodybuilding contest.

→ Gigi Rodriguez, age 46, lost 47 pounds of fat and built 7 pounds of muscle.

→ Robin Parr, age 65, lost 56 pounds of fat and built 8 pounds of muscle.

Overall, the program under Lydia's command seemed to be in good hands. I was standing to the side, watching Lydia direct the meeting, and I counted 49 people seated in front of her. When it was time for questions, Lydia answered each one correctly with skill. I was impressed.

Then I noticed that three of our best 2012 subjects—Angel Rodriguez, Melissa Norman, and Boyd Welsch—were seated among the group. Later I learned that Angel had motivated four people to get involved, Melissa had inspired three more to join the program, and Boyd had influenced at least five people. Almost every new person had been motivated and even mentored by participants from my original May 2012 group of 44 subjects.

I had mentored Lydia, who in turn had mentored dozens of participants, who were now mentoring even more trainees. It was infectious. As on the Internet, the Body Fat Breakthrough participation had gone viral.

Lydia had an amazing influence on recruiting overweight women and men to join the Breakthrough program. Part of her success was based on her ability to connect and inspire. She knew how to connect through listening, understanding, and forging coalitions. Then she inspired her trainees by encouraging them with a sense of shared purpose. It worked well for her. In fact, I've observed that many of her mentored subjects have applied the same connect-and-inspire techniques to their daily lives.

Lydia has positively influenced many Breakthrough participants, and these trainees have turned around and influenced their friends.

CIRCLE OF INFLUENCE

Within Gainesville Health & Fitness, on a wall next to the main strength-training area, are 5-foot-tall photographs of four of our best before-and-after Breakthrough subjects. Below these almost-life-size images are smaller photos of 10 participants.

This before-and-after photo exhibit was assembled in January 2013, and it's the most eye-catching and influential display I've ever seen in a health club. Members stop, stare, point, ask questions, and often want to join the program immediately.

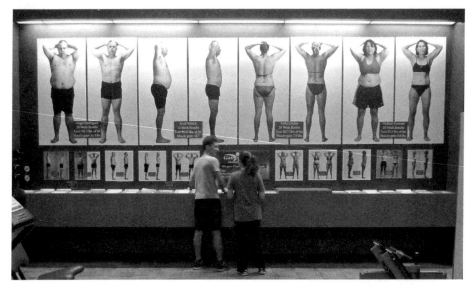

The full-color before-and-after photos on display at Gainesville Health & Fitness challenge members to "Tap the Muscle-Building Power of Negative Training and Lose Up to 30 Pounds in 30 Days."

Some of the individuals on the wall have become regional celebrities. Angel Rodriguez and Storm Roberts were featured on local TV stations and discussed their fat-loss experiences, and they are recognized throughout the Gainesville area. One attractive 21-year-old woman on the wall has had to change her cell phone number twice.

In case you haven't noticed, your brand-new body carries with it influencing possibilities. You now have a soapbox to stand on. Like Lydia Maree, Boyd Welsch, and others, you'll have a chance to offer meaningful guidelines to influence others on losing fat.

I hope that you'll take this role seriously and help lead people in the right direction.

A Strong, Lean Body . . . Permanently!

To keep your body permanently strong and lean, you must have the discipline to apply Fat Bombs 1 through 10, not only for 6 weeks or 12 weeks, but for the rest of your life.

The Fat Bombs, or guidelines, that I've challenged you with are seldom glamorous and sometimes hard to face. But practicing them, as you have been doing, leads eventually to the lifestyle changes that must occur for year-to-year permanence.

Building muscle to lose fat . . . This is the critical principle that I've spent more than 50 years applying, researching, and—with negative-accentuated training—perfecting. My Breakthrough manual supplies everything you need to build muscle to lose fat.

Extra muscle will not only help you lose more fat but will also make your body harder, firmer, tighter, and better looking. Again, examine the comparison photos within. Every one of my 145 subjects who trained in 2012 added significant muscle to his or her body. There was not a single person—male or female, young or old—who registered a problem with the development of larger, stronger muscle.

In fact, it was just the opposite. Muscle proved to be a friend, savior, and liberator.

Persist and Prevail

In conclusion, you should now know that muscle is a vital aspect of maintaining your leanness. The negative-training applications described in this book are your ***personal breakthrough*** to a great-looking body, physical preservation, and an enhanced life.

With science, preparation, and consistency you can:

Stay strong and remain lean for the rest of your life.

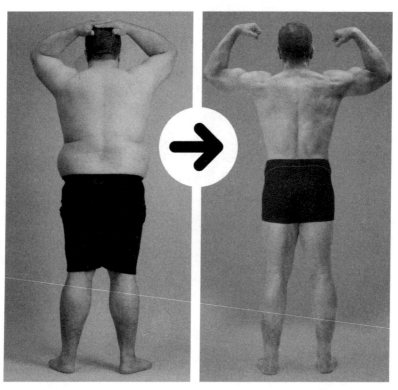

The Introduction of this book opened with before-and-after photos of Angel Rodriguez, who lost 121 pounds of fat. It seems appropriate to close with the backside shots of Angel. These photos show clearly that he also built more than 20 pounds of muscle. My concluding challenge to Angel and to you is this:

Apply, adapt, persist, and prevail.

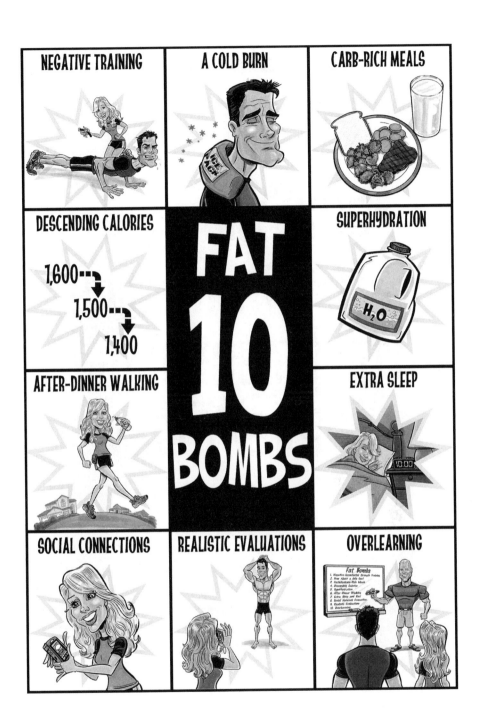

X-Force™: Innovative Strength-Training Equipment of the Future, *Today*

X-FORCE is a new fitness-equipment system manufactured in Stockholm, Sweden, that has been developed to make negative-accentuated exercise simpler and more effective. I have been involved with X-Force as a paid consultant since 2009, doing research on the machines and writing historical and instructional material for the company.

As you've learned in this book, heavy negative-accentuated resistance allows the lifter to work at more intense effort levels, which research shows translates into greater strength and muscle gains in less time. X-Force machines facilitate this method of training using a patented "tilting" weight stack that creates 40 percent heavier resistance on the negative, or eccentric (lowering), part of the exercise.

A set on an X-Force machine provides a precise, measurable, and progressive overload of negative resistance. One key benefit of X-Force is that each set can be safely performed solo, without a spotter, because the machine essentially lightens the load during the positive part of the lift. Much of the uniqueness of X-Force machines involves the tilting weight stack. At the bottom of the weight stack, an electric servomotor powers the tilt. The lifter pushes a blue button, which moves the weight stack into the vertical position. Once in position, the blue button flashes, indicating that you can pull the selector pin and place an appropriate amount of resistance on the weight stack. The resistance is noted in kilograms on the left side and pounds on the right. Important: The resistance that you select is for the negative phase of the exercises.

Included with the motor is a sensor that recognizes movement in either direction. At a 45-degree angle, during the positive phase, the resistance on the machine weighs significantly less. The exerciser lifts the resistance in 3 seconds to the top position and pauses. In the vertical position, during the negative phase, the resistance weighs 40 percent more than during the positive phase. The lifter then lowers the resistance slowly for 5 seconds and continues exercising this way for 4 to 8 repetitions, or until the negative phase can no longer be completed.

For a beginning trainee, a routine includes only one set of six to eight X-Force machines. A workout is finished in 20 minutes or less. X-Force, properly performed, provides deep muscular stimulation in minimum time. Plenty of rest is required for complete recovery.

You're probably wondering, "Where can I work out on X-Force machines?"

Unfortunately, unless you live in Europe; Gainesville, Florida; or near Philadelphia, you won't be able to take advantage of these unique training machines (although, as you've learned in this book, you can still apply the principles of negative-accentuated lifting very effectively with free weights, machines, or your own body weight).

At least a dozen training facilities in Europe are using X-Force machines. In the United States, currently there are only two places you'll find prototype X-Force machines: Joe Cirulli's Gainesville Health & Fitness, which hosted my Body Fat Breakthrough program participants, and Roger Schwab's Main Line Health & Fitness in Bryn Mawr, Pennsylvania.

Soon, however, you will start seeing X-Force equipment in the United

States, and I expect that most major health clubs and gyms will sport X-Force machines within the next decade. Meanwhile, here's a sneak peek at X-Force and how it works. Pictured are the six most popular X-Force machines, photographed at Main Line Health & Fitness, where personal instructors trained more than 600 people exclusively on the machines in 2012. To see videos of the equipment in action, visit Main Line Health & Fitness's Web site MLHF.com.

Leg Press: This machine targets the lower body's major muscles: gluteals, hamstrings, and quadriceps. At the position pictured, the trainee is near the turnaround of the positive motion. As the weight stack tilts, the negative phase begins and the involved muscles are stressed with 40 percent more resistance.

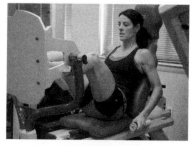

Leg Press

Pec Seated Press: Since most trainees are familiar with the bench press, the Pec Seated Press immediately, from the first full repetition, draws attention to the negative phase, perhaps better than any other X-Force machine. The individual in the photo has just experienced the positive turnaround to the negative, and he feels the resistance intensely in his pectoral and triceps muscles.

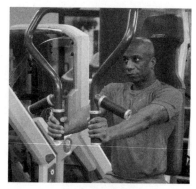

Pec Seated Press

Lat Back Circular: This pulling exercise allows more than 200 degrees of rotation of the shoulders and involves the largest and strongest upper-body muscles, the latissimus dorsi. The trainee is near the negative-to-positive turnaround.

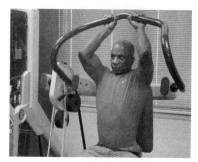

Lat Back Circular

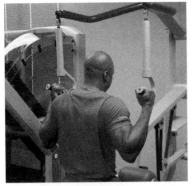

Lat Back Pull

Lat Back Pull: This is a downward-exerting movement for the biceps and latissimus dorsi muscles. In some routines, the Lat Back Pull is used immediately after the Lat Back Circular, which allows the biceps to force the latissimus dorsi to a deeper level of fatigue.

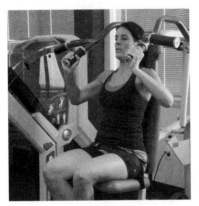

Deltoid Press

Deltoid Press: This pressing sequence works both the deltoids and triceps. Once the resistance is pushed overhead, the weight stack tilts, and instantly there's a 40 percent overload on the negative.

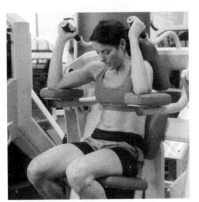

Abdominal Crunch

Abdominal Crunch: When performing what is often the last exercise in a routine, it's important to pull with the abdominal muscles—and not the arms. The trainee pauses briefly in the crunched position, feels the negative transfer, lowers the resistance slowly until the weight stack touches, and repeats for the appropriate repetitions.

Factory Fitness in Sweden

Norrkoping, Sweden, with a population of 140,000, is approximately 100 miles south of Stockholm. Near the center of Norrkoping is one of the largest and best-equipped fitness clubs in the world, a 57,000-square-foot facility called Factory Fitness.

Besides having the typical equipment and physical activities, such as treadmills, Spin bikes, Step machines, free weights, kickboxing, group exercising, and various dance classes, Factory Fitness features the largest array of X-Force machines anywhere. There are 112 X-Force machines in four color-coded sections designated for beginners, advanced athletes, seniors, and people specifically interested in weight loss.

Factory Fitness is owned and operated by Peter Ericsson, who has developed clubs throughout Sweden since 1987. Ericsson's Factory Fitness also serves as a showroom for X-Force equipment. This large-scale gym of the future is in operation today in Norrkoping, Sweden.

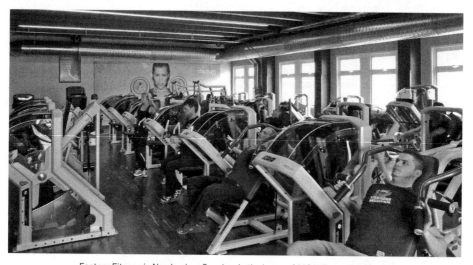

Factory Fitness in Norrkoping, Sweden, is the home of 112 X-Force machines.

For more information about X-Force, visit X-Force.se.

Gainesville Health & Fitness in Florida

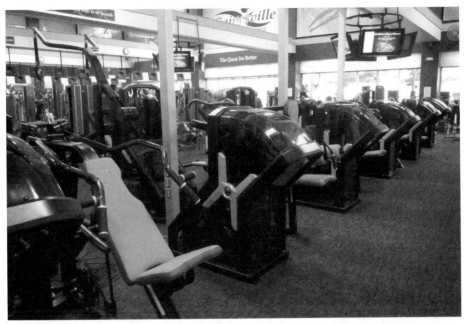

At one end of the main floor of Gainesville Health & Fitness are 14 X-Force machines, which are divided into two back-to-back lines.

Joe Cirulli's X-Force machines are housed in two lines on the main floor of his facility, where they are available to all club members.

Cirulli is currently adding 12,000 square feet to his club's floor plan, and in 2014 the facility will have an enclosed training area for two complete lines of X-Force equipment that can be used for 6-week programs of my Body Fat Breakthrough.

The staff at GHF appreciate that negative-accentuated training, by stimulating and directing the body's natural hormones, provides an important new way to build muscle and lose fat. The members are excited about being in the forefront of the negative-accentuated reform.

Again, if you are ever in the Gainesville area, you are invited to visit GHF, 4820 Newberry Road, Gainesville, FL 32607, for an X-Force demonstration and trial.

Be prepared for the new era in strength training.

BIBLIOGRAPHY

Ainesworth, B. E., and others. "Compendium of Physical Activities: An Update of Activity Codes and MET Intensities," *Medicine and Science in Sports and Exercise* 32 (Supplement): S498–S516, 2000.

Boschmann, Michael, and others. "Water-Induced Thermogenesis," *Journal of Clinical Endocrinology & Metabolism* 88: 6015–6019, 2003.

Cermak, N. M., and others. "Eccentric Exercise Increases Satellite Cell Content in Type II Muscle Fibers," *Medicine and Science in Sports and Exercise* 45: 230–237, 2013.

Colvin, Robert H., and Olson, Susan C. *Keeping It Off: Winning at Weight Loss.* New York: Simon & Schuster, 1985.

Davis, J. Mark, and others. "Weight Control and Calorie Expenditure: Thermogenesis Effects of Pre-Prandial Exercise," *Addictive Behaviors* 14:347–351, 1989.

Forbes, Gilbert. "The Adult Decline in Lean Body Mass," *Human Biology* 48: 161–173, 1976.

Heller, H. Craig, and Grahn, Dennis A. "Enhancing Thermal Exchange in Humans and Practical Applications," *Disruptive Science and Technology* 1: 1–10, 2012.

Jackowski, Edward J. *Hold It! You're Exercising Wrong.* New York: Fireside, 1995.

Jones, Arthur. "Accentuate the Negative," *IronMan*: 32: 30, 31, 56–59, January 1973.

Komi, P. V., and Buskirk, E. R. "Effect of Eccentric and Concentric Muscle Conditioning on Tension and Electrical Activity in Human Muscle," *Ergonomics* 15: 417-434, 1972.

Knight, Bob, with Hammel, Bob. *The Power of Negative Thinking.* New York: Houghton Mifflin Harcourt, 2013.

Madison, Deborah. *Vegetarian Cooking for Everyone*, Tenth Anniversary Edition. New York: Broadway Books, 2007.

Norrbrand, L., and others. "Resistance Training Using Eccentric Overload Induces Early Adaptations in Skeletal Muscle Size," *European Journal of Applied Physiology* 102: 271-281, 2008.

Pedersen, B.K., and Fabbraio, M.A. "Muscle as an Endocrine Organ: Focus on Muscle-Derived Interleukin-6," *Physiological Reviews* 88: 1379-1406, 2008

Pollock, M. L., and others. "Measurement of Cardiorespiratory Fitness and Body Composition in the Clinical Setting," *Comprehensive Therapy* 6: 12-27, 1980.

Roig, M., and others. "The Effects of Eccentric Versus Concentric Resistance Training on Muscle Strength and Mass in Healthy Adults: A Systematic Review with Meta-Analyses," *British Journal of Sports Medicine*: 43: 556-568, 2009.

Schoenfeld, Brad. "The Mechanisms of Muscle Hypertrophy and Their Application to Resistance Training," *Journal of Strength and Conditioning Research* 24: 2857-2872, 2010.

ACKNOWLEDGMENTS

Sincere thanks goes to the following people who helped me in the *Body Fat Breakthrough* research and book project:

Mats Thulin from Stockholm, Sweden, for rejuvenating my decades-old negative-training interest after I used his X-Force machines for the first time in 2008.

The staff of Gainesville Health & Fitness for welcoming the X-Force machines into their facility in 2012 and then working synergistically with me throughout my research project.

Lydia Maree for her enduring work in organizing, supervising, and training test subjects and for her continued programming and follow-up at Gainesville Health & Fitness.

Jim Lennon for his computer skills in handouts, record keeping, and measurement results.

Glen Purdy for his expertise in "getting the word out" at Gainesville Health & Fitness.

Mindy Miller for her before-and-after photography.

Ted Spiker for his input in the preparation of my book proposal.

Keelan Parham of Orlando, Florida, for his Fat Bomb illustrations and inside-the-body drawings.

David Ponsonby and **Barbara Creighton** for their valuable suggestions after reviewing my book manuscript.

Jeanenne Darden for not only helping me throughout the entire project, but for her devotion to our children and home while I made my weekly trips to and from Gainesville Health & Fitness for more than a year. Thank you, Jeanenne, for allowing me extra time in my office, which you designed. It is a frequent reminder to me of our success as a team.

Jeff Csatari, executive editor of *Men's Health* and *Women's Health* books at Rodale for improving the text as only an experienced editor can with enthusiasm, skill, and insight, especially from the reader's point of view.

Amy King and **Mike Smith** of Rodale for their impressive design and art direction.

Roger Schwab of Bryn Mawr, Pennsylvania, for his negative-training knowledge and his overall encouragement.

Michael Spillane of Gainesville, Florida, for his genuine friendship.

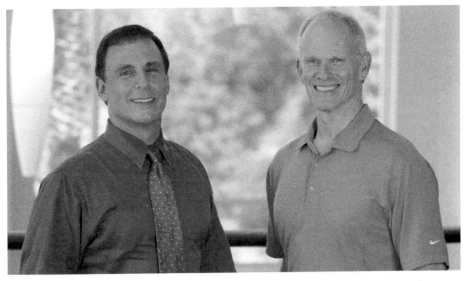

I first visited Joe Cirulli at his Gainesville club in 1980. His large membership numbers, as well as the way he organized his exercise instruction, amazed me. Cirulli was agreeable to doing fat-loss and muscle-building studies with selected groups of his fitness-minded people. Over the next three decades, I measured, trained, and dieted many test subjects and used their before-and-after photos in 14 books. The Breakthrough book was my most challenging body-transformation project to date and success would not have been possible without Joe Cirulli's commitment to excellence.

Joe, for the record, you and Gainesville Health & Fitness are # 1 in service and # 1 in results. Thank you for pushing people to do their best . . . and thank you for promoting the positive in the negative.

INDEX

Underscored page references indicate boxed text and tables.
Boldface references indicate photographs and illustrations.

Abdominal crunch, 162–63, **163**
   X-Force, 309, **309**
Achong-Coan, Roxanne, 73
   body transformation of, **70**
Actin, in muscle, 90
Aerobics
   ineffectiveness of, 97
   for maintenance of new body, 277
   misconception about, 95
After-dinner walking. *See* Walking, after-dinner
Aging, muscle atrophy and, 19
Alcohol, avoiding, 177, 193, 256
Anti-inflammatory drugs, 92
Appetite control, water for, 190
Apps, for weight-loss support, 212
Arm routines, extremely slow repetitions in, 68
Arm size, increasing, 294, **295**
Aromas, added to meals, 258
Assertiveness, 216
Atkins diet, 176

Back raise, 132–33, **133**
Backslides, recovering from, 216, 259, 276
Bagels, 282
Baldwin, Cris, body transformation of, **180**
Barbell bench press, 134–35, **135**
Barbell curl, 138–39, **139**
Barbell overhead press, 140–41, **141**
Barbells. *See also* Free weights
   misconceptions about, 89
   problems of slow training with, 69
   2-4 negative training with, 82–83
Barbell shoulder shrug, 144–45, **145**
Barbell squat, 136–37, **137**
Basic Four Food Groups, 175, 177
Basic Seven Food Groups, 177
Bernhard, Anya, body transformation of, **215, 244**
Beverages
   alcoholic, 177, 193, 256
   types to avoid, 193
   water as (*see* Superhydration; Water)
Biceps Curl, X-Force, 63–64, 86, 87, **105**
Bigger Arms in 2 Weeks course, 294, **295**
Black and blue marks, 283
Black bears
   brown fat in, 36

   heat dissipation in, 31, 33, 168
Body composition, water in, 188
Body fat
   calculating percentage of, 96
   calorie cutting promoting, 4
   composition of, 94
   corresponding to skin-fold thickness, 226
   cortisol and, 206, 207, 208
   from creeping obesity, 20
   cross-section appearance of, 91, **91**
   effect on muscle function, 19
   functions of, 94–95
   ideal percentage of, 225
   locations of, 5
   loss of (*see* Fat loss)
   measuring, 5 (*see also* Skin-fold measurements)
   metabolic rate of, 21
   regained after dieting, 3–4
   stressors contributing to, 207
   types of, 5, 94
Body Fat Breakthrough program
   assessing current condition before starting, 221–28
   commitment to, 6–7, 265
   continuing, after 6 weeks, 264–68
   importance of mentoring in, 301–2
   partner for, 215–16, 259
   physician approval for, 222
   preparing for, 228–31
   recovering from backslides in, 216, 259, 276
   results from
      determining, 261, 264
      expected, x, xi
   rules for following, 57
   simplicity of, 6–7, 43, 292–93
   test panelists in
      requirements of, 39–40
      results of, 5–6, 23–26, **25**, 40–43, **42**, 228, 264 (*see also* Body transformations)
   social network for, 211–12
Body Fat Breakthrough Workout Card, 249, 249
Body-part measurements chart, 224
Body Solid machines, 116, 152
Body transformations, xi, **25, 42**
   Achong-Coan, Roxanne, **70**
   Baldwin, Cris, **180**
   Bernhard, Anya, **215, 244**